New Ideas on the Structure of
the Nervous System in
Man and Vertebrates

New Ideas on the Structure of the Nervous System in Man and Vertebrates

Santiago Ramón y Cajal

translated from the French
by Neely Swanson and Larry W. Swanson

A Bradford Book
The MIT Press
Cambridge, Massachusetts
London, England

This work was originally published in French as *Les Nouvelles idées sur la structure du système nerveux chez l'homme et chez les vertebrés*, translated from Spanish by L. Azoulay and reviewed and augmented by the author, by C. Reinwald & Cie., Paris, 1894.

This book was set in Palatino by DEKR Corporation and printed and bound in the United States of America.

Library of Congress Cataloging-in-Publication Data

Ramón y Cajal, Santiago, 1852–1934.
  [Textura del sistema nervioso del hombre y de los vertebrados. English]
  New ideas on the structure of the nervous system in man and vertebrates / by Santiago Ramón y Cajal translated from the French by Neely Swanson and Larry W. Swanson.
      p.   cm.
  Translation of: Les nouvelle idées sur la structure du système nerveux chez l'homme et chez les vertebrés (which was a translation from the Spanish).
  Includes bibliographical references.
  ISBN 0-262-03166-3
  1. Nervous system—Histology. 2. Neuroanatomy. I. Title.
  [DNLM: 1. Nervous System—anatomy & histology. 2. Nervous System-
-ultrastructure.   WL   101 R175t]
QM575.R343   1990
611'.8—dc20
DNLM/DLC
for Library of Congress   90-5690
                                                                    CIP

Contents

Translator's Foreword

> . . . living nature, far from being drained and exhausted, keeps back from all of us, great and small, immeasurable stretches of unknown territory; . . . even in the regions apparently most worked over, there remain still many unknown things to be cleared up.[1]

Today's revolution in biological thought spawned by molecular genetics was preceded by an equally exciting period in the 1880s, when the work of Pasteur, Koch, and Lister gave rise to the field of microbiology. At that time, many of the best minds in medical research shifted their attention from the study of cells first undertaken by Schwann and Virchow to the much tinier organisms that infect them, just as attention now focuses even more narrowly on the genetic material that controls life itself. Against this background, it is not surprising to find Santiago Ramón y Cajal, then a 33-year-old professor of anatomy in Zaragosa, commissioned by the government to study the Spanish cholera epidemic of 1885. With characteristic rigor and imagination, he established the presence of the *bacillus* identified by Koch in India two years earlier and even devised the first useful animal vaccine based on injections of heat-inactivated cultures of the bacteria.

Despite this success, which the local government rewarded with the gift of a magnificent Zeiss microscope, Cajal's future lay elsewhere. While in Madrid in 1887 to examine candidates for professorships in anatomy, he visited his old friend Si-

1. Cajal, S. Ramón y. *Recollections of My Life,* translated by E. H. Craigie with the assistance of J. Cano. Cambridge, MA: The MIT Press, 1989, 279.

marro, who had just returned from studying in Paris, to see
first-hand the latest histological preparations developed
abroad. Cajal had recently taken it upon himself to prepare a
histology textbook based on original observations and illustra-
tions, since no such work had been produced in Spain. It was
on this occasion, at 41 Calle del Arco de Santa Maria, that
Cajal first saw preparations of the nervous system stained with
the Golgi method; it was an event that galvanized his scientific
life and led to the most profound body of work by a single
investigator in the long history of neuroscience—a history that
can be traced back to the writings of Aristotle.

In the absence of a definitive history of modern neuroscience
Cajal's autobiography provides the best, and certainly the
most entertaining, account of his work as well as the sociology
of nineteenth-century science in general. As he points out,
neurologists of the time entertained the somewhat romantic
view that a detailed understanding of brain structure was of
the utmost importance for building a rational psychology.
However, the methods available were woefully inadequate for
establishing the morphology of most nerve cells; it was simply
not possible to determine the origin and termination of nerve
fibers or the way in which one cell connects with another.

The excitement engendered by the Golgi preparations led
Cajal to abandon what he thought might have been a sure
path to fame and fortune in bacteriology for what he considered an absolute path to poverty—and happiness—in the mod-
est science of histology, the "religion of the cell." In 1887 he
assumed the Chair of Histology in Barcelona and devoted
tremendous energy to exploring the Golgi method. Although
Golgi had introduced it in 1873 and had published a magnificent book describing his research in 1886,[2] the method had
not excited much interest outside of Italy because the number
and kinds of cells that were impregnated often varied considerably in different experiments, and the great researchers of

2. Golgi, C. *Sulla Fina Anatomia degli Organi Centrali del Sistema Nervoso.* Milan
Hoepli, 1886.

the time favored the application of techniques they themselves had developed. Cajal's own strategy consisted of improving the reliability of the method itself (resulting in the double-impregnation procedure), and applying ordinary common sense, as he called it, to the problem of brain structure. The great advantage of the Golgi method, of course, is that only a small proportion of the nerve cells in any particular piece of tissue are stained; Cajal saw that to simplify the problem even further, it would be advantageous to examine simpler, smaller animals (neurologists at the time favored human material) as well as embryonic material. Instead of examining the impenetrable, full-grown forest, Cajal decided to begin in the nursery stage with the young trees and follow their growth.

By Cajal's own account 1888 was his greatest year, his year of fortune: it was then that he discovered the laws governing the morphology and connections of nerve cells in the gray matter, first in the cerebellum, then in the retina, and then systematically in many other parts of the nervous system. He worked with a fury; annoyed by the slowness of the press, he started and published his own journal, the *Revista trimestral de Histologia normal y pathológica,* that reported his discoveries. In 1890 alone he published fourteen original papers on the nervous system, including the discovery of the growth cone.

Despite an obscure background his fame grew quickly, particularly under the influence of the German master Koelliker. By 1894 he had published the review that is translated here, which summarized his revolutionary view of the nervous system (see appendices A & B for a history of this book's evolution). This small work was important for two main reasons. First, it reviewed the scientific evidence favoring the neuron doctrine and Cajal's concept of dynamic polarity for a wide audience. Cajal claimed that axons end freely in the gray matter, where they contact the dendrites and cell bodies of other nerve cells. Together the dendrites and cell body form the receptive part in the chain of conduction, and nerve impulses are transmitted by way of axons that contact other cells, rather than being continuous with them. This was in stark contrast to the widely held views of Gerlach and Golgi that the nervous system forms a cellular reticulum, a concept that rendered the structure of individual neurons or groups of neurons irrelevant because under such conditions the pathways followed by nerve impulses would be indeterminant. According to Golgi, dendrites served a strictly nutritive role in neuronal function, whereas the axons formed an interconnected reticulum.

The second reason this book is of interest is that it presents in embryonic form the basic plan Cajal followed in the publication of his monumental survey of vertebrate neurohistology, published in Spanish as three volumes between 1897 and 1903,[3] and later expanded and published in French between 1909 and 1911.[4] The French edition is unparalleled in its scope, accuracy, and insight and is unquestionably the most important book ever published in neuroanatomy. Nevertheless, it was through the new ideas summarized in the present volume that Cajal won the Nobel prize in Medicine in 1906, together with his scientific rival Golgi. The occasion of this award was particularly interesting from a historical point of view because two distinguished scientists, using essentially the same methods, arrived at and articulated diametrically opposed conclusions about the basic organization of the nervous system.[5] It was not until the advent of electron microscopy that the last serious adherents of Golgi's reticular theory admitted defeat.

The pace of Cajal's work never slowed; he continued to make numerous contributions of the first rank to the fields of neuronal plasticity, invertebrate neurohistology, and many others; he also published books on color photography, advice to young investigators, and the philosophical observations of

3. Cajal, S. Ramón y. *Textura del sistema nervioso del hombre y de los vertebrados* (3 volumenes) Madrid, 1897, 1899 y 1904.

4. Cajal, S. Ramón y. *Histology du Système Nerveux de l'Homme et des Vertébrés.* Vols. I and II. Paris: Maloine. Reprinted Madrid, Consejo Superior de Investigaciones Cientificas, 1952.

5. *Nobel Lectures: Physiology and Medicine,* 1901–1921. Amsterdam, Elsevier, 1967, pp. 185–256.

an octogenarian. He even published a series of popular articles under the pen name of Doctor Bacteria!

This great man died on October 17, 1934, at the age of 82; he was buried in Madrid's Necropolis alongside his beloved wife. As a measure of his great esteem in Spain, the funeral was attended by representatives of all classes of society, from the aristocracy to the workers.

Readers interested in further exploring Cajal's life, research, and the times he lived in may consult several biographies.[6] However, the most fascinating source of information about Cajal is his own writings.[7] In preparing this translation, we have tried to preserve as much of the original style as possible in modern English. In line with this, we have, for example, taken the liberty of substituting dorsal for anterior and ventral for posterior where appropriate, and have often substituted a modern anatomical term for a nineteenth-century term after Cajal introduced the older term for the first time. All footnotes in the text are those found in the 1894 edition, with the exception of that on p. 174, which we added for the sake of clarity. We hope that readers will enjoy reading this brilliant work as much as we enjoyed translating it.

In closing, we would especially like to thank Jeremy Norman, Charles Stevens, Jim Cox, and Fiona Stevens for their valuable contributions to this translation.

Larry W. Swanson
La Jolla, California
July 1989

6.   Cannon, D. F. *Explorer of the Human Brain. The Life of Santiago Ramón y Cajal.* New York: Schuman, 1949. Albarracin, A. *Santiago Ramón y Cajal o la Pasión de España.* Barcelona: Editorial Labor, 1982. DeFilipe, J. and E.G. Jones. *Cajal on the Cerebral Cortex.* New York: Oxford University Press, 1988. Williams, H. *Don Quixote of the Microscope.* London: Jonathan Cape, 1954.
7.   As well as the works cited above, see: Cajal, S. Ramón y. *Degeneration and Regeneration of the Nervous System.* Translated and edited by R. M. May. London: Oxford University Press, 2 vols., 1928.

New Ideas on the Structure of
the Nervous System in
Man and Vertebrates

Introduction

A thorough understanding of the structure of the nervous system clearly provides an essential foundation for the disciplines of physiology and pathology. The nervous system mediates dynamic interactions between widely separate parts of the organism and regulates all cellular activities, with the ultimate goal of conserving the life of the individual as well as the species. However, it is also clear that no other system is plagued with such a broad range of problems that have been studied with so little success, despite the great importance its understanding has from the anatomical, physiological, and pathological points of view.

The simple problem of nerve cell shape is only now on the verge of being solved, despite the fact that the morphology of cells in most other tissues has been known for some time.

Our lack of understanding is due to several major difficulties encountered in analyzing the nervous system. The cells of the brain and spinal cord are often quite large, and their thin processes, which branch repeatedly, are interwoven within the gray matter. The complexity of this dense feltwork has defied attempts to follow individual elements and establish how they end.

One can only begin to appreciate the forbidding complexity of the gray matter and the technical difficulties that must be solved to shed even one ray of light on this otherwise dark terrain, when the many fine processes of neuroglial cells and nerve fibers from other centers are added; when the fact that all of these elements are held together by a small amount of very effective interstitial cement is taken into account and when it is realized that nerve cells are quite delicate and subject to alteration.

However, despite all of these obstacles, the problem is of such pressing interest that many anatomists and physiologists have devoted themselves to clarifying the morphology and connections of nerve cells.

Progress in each era of research has been based on the use of a particular analytical method. Gerlach introduced the carmine staining method that allowed Deiters to distinguish two distinct classes of processes arising from nerve cells, and to establish the morphology of glial cells. Türck, Bouchard, Fleschig, Charcot, and others applied the secondary degeneration method to study the course of axons to nerve centers. And Fleschig introduced an equally informative approach based on the fact that each fiber bundle undergoes myelination at a particular time during development, thus allowing the temporal pattern of myelination to be followed in the embryo.

Nevertheless these methods, as well as others based on the selective staining of axons or myelin by osmic acid (Exner's method), gold chloride (Freud's method), or hematoxyline (Weigert's method), have not clarified the most important questions: how do the processes of nerve cells end? How do axons coursing through the white matter end?

The only thing that was known about these problems before the work of the Italian school was based on the results of Deiters, Wagner, Koelliker, Krause, and others. Namely, all of the ganglion cells in nerve centers display two kinds of processes: one consists of a number of thick, highly branched *protoplasmic* or *dendritic* processes, while the other is thinner, has a smooth contour, and extends as a nerve fiber called the axon or Deiters' process.

To explain intercellular communication, it was presumed that anastomoses between dendrites form a thick, continuous plexus in the gray matter. With regard to the origin of nerves, it was considered established that the motor nerves represent simple extensions of Deiters' processes, whereas the sensory nerves arise from fibers of the interstitial dendritic plexus.

Figure 1 graphically illustrates this point of view, which has dominated scientific thought for more than thirty years.

This state of affairs would still prevail if the illustrious Italian scholar Golgi had not developed an analytical method that was superior to all others. When a small piece of the brain or spinal cord that has been fixed in potassium dichromate is immersed in silver nitrate for twenty-four hours, an opaque red precipitate forms selectively in a small number of elements in the gray matter, differentiating them with the greatest clarity and yielding an extraordinarily beautiful pattern in which the finest details of the thinnest cellular processes can be seen. With the valuable help of this method, Golgi succeeded in proving two very important points.

First, every nerve cell has an axon, which, like the dendrites, gives rise to many thin collateral branches. And second, the dendrites do not form a plexus, but instead branch many times and end freely.

With regard to the way in which cells and fibers are connected, Golgi was still influenced by Gerlach's reticular theory, although he believed that the reticulum consists of the intermingled collaterals and terminal branches of nerve fibers or axons, rather than of dendrites; he maintained the reservation that this axonal plexus should be regarded as nothing more than an anatomical hypothesis. In a sense, the cell body and dendrites were removed from participation in the transmission of neural impulses; thus, according to Golgi, they play a strictly nutritive role.

As I shall demonstrate later, the Italian histologist was unable to break entirely with tradition. As early as 1885, certain histologists had raised the possibility that nerve fibers and axons end freely like dendrites, and His and Forel both supported this doctrine. His' view was based on embryological studies that invariably showed neuroblasts as independent elements before the production of dendrites, and Forel's opinion was based on negative evidence in so far as he had never observed the slightest trace of an interstitial axonal plexus in the gray matter. Nevertheless, both His and Forel were unable

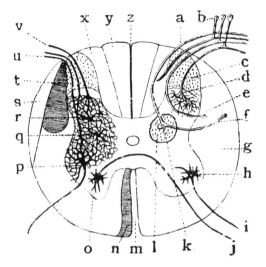

Figure 1
Connections of the ventral and dorsal roots of the spinal cord according to the older theory. Compare with figure 4.

a: dorsal root fiber that arises from a cell in Clarke's column; *b*: unipolar cells of the spinal ganglia; *d*: root fiber ending in the reticulum of the dorsal horn; *e*: root fiber that courses longitudinally across the lateral funiculus; *f*: fiber coursing from Clarke's column to the lateral funiculus; *g*: lateral funiculus; *h*: root or motor cell that gives rise to fiber *i*; *j*: ventral root fiber from cell *o* in the ventral horn on the opposite side; *k*: Clarke's column; *m*: ventral fissure of the spinal cord; *n*: ventral bundle of the descending pyramidal tract (Türck's bundle); *p*: ventral horn cell whose dendrites form a plexus; *q*: region where the dorsal root fibers also end; *r*: cells in the dorsal horn with dendrites contributing to the plexus; *s*: ascending bundle of the lateral funiculus (cerebellar pathway); *t*: lateral bundle of the pyramidal tract; *u, v*: dorsal root fibers ending in a plexus; *x*: Burdach's tract; *y*: Goll's tract; *z*: dorsal sulcus of the spinal cord.

to demonstrate the terminal arborizations of axons, or the way that they establish connections with nerve cells. This is where I succeeded in the brain, spinal cord, olfactory bulb, retina, optic centers, sympathetic system, and elsewhere, demonstrating beyond doubt the way nerve fibers end. My ideas, which were somewhat speculative at the time I had the honor of publishing them, have since come to be regarded as scientific fact. Thus, a number of recent monographs by Koelliker, His, Lenhossék, van Gehuchten, and Retzius, as well as those of my brother and Claudio Sala, have confirmed and extended my work and have revealed new and important structural arrangements as well.[1] Thus, I believe that the time is now ripe to outline our current state of knowledge about the structure of the nervous system, concentrating on the basic facts and results that may be considered firmly established.

1. My results with the silver chromate-sublimate method on the spinal cord, brain, cerebellum, medulla, Ammon's horn, and retina of the human infant, lamb, horse, and cow have allowed me to verify the accuracy of the following descriptions. I should add that the structural figures accompanying the text, which appear highly schematic, are in fact *less* so than the actual preparations.—AZOULAY.

Chapter 1
The Spinal Cord

Golgi's work shed light on many aspects of spinal cord neurophysiology, extending and confirming a great deal of earlier knowledge. Ideas about this medullary structure may be summarized as follows.

The white matter was thought to consist of the axons of cells in the gray matter that converge after initially coursing transversely and then turning to run longitudinally.

Two regions were distinguished in the gray matter. The *ventral horn* was thought to contain cells (Golgi motor cells) with a long axon that either entered the ventral root or contributed to the ventrolateral funiculus, while a majority of the cells in the *dorsal horn* (Golgi sensory cells) were thought to generate a thin axon that branched many times and then lost its individuality. Instead of entering the white matter, this axon became part of the interstitial plexus described by Golgi in the gray matter.

It had been known since the work of Ranvier, Lenhossék, His, and others that dorsal roots constitute the central branches of a single bifurcating process arising from individual spinal ganglion cells. After entering the gray matter, they were thought to ramify and anastomose with the collaterals of axons from motor cells in the ventral horn, thus establishing the sensory-motor arc, the normal pathway underlying reflexes.

After reaching the level of the spinal cord, sensory impressions would thus be forced to traverse the gray matter reticulum, where links would be established between the terminal branches of dorsal root fibers and the collaterals of ventral root fibers. In this view, summarized in figures 1 and 2A, the dendrites of neurons play no role in conduction.

My own studies on the spinal cord began near the end of 1888. However, before starting research on this particular problem, I had studied the cerebellum of embryonic birds and mammals. The results of this work were considerably different from those presented in Golgi's diagrams with regard to the morphology of nerve cells and the connections between fibers, and led me to ideas about the structure of nerve centers that are much more consistent with observable facts. These studies demonstrated the following:

> 1. Nerve cells are independent units whose dendrites and axons never form anastomoses.
> 2. Every axon ends by way of flexuous, varicose arborizations like the ramifications of nerve fibers at muscle end plates.
> 3. These arborizations are applied to the cell body or dendrites of neurons where connections are formed by way of contiguity or contact, an arrangement that transmits current as effectively as connections established by way of continuity.
> 4. The cell body as well as the dendrites play a role in conduction, not just nutrition.

Our examination of the spinal cord was simplified greatly by the application of these new principles about the general morphology of nerve cells. And, if I could rely on the law of structural unity, which holds that a particular tissue has a uniform structure throughout, then there was reason to hope that the same basic organization would be found in the spinal cord and the cerebellum. My foresight was rewarded: the spinal cord can be viewed as a small brain that is reversed in the sense that white matter is concentrated around the periphery rather than in the center.

White Matter
Studies in the embryo and newborn animal are easier to carry out because the elements are shorter, and the gray matter and

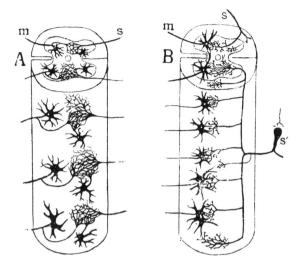

Figure 2
A: Golgi's view of the communication between ventral and dorsal roots. *m*:
ventral root fiber; *s*: dorsal root fiber with collaterals that form a plexus in the
gray matter with the recurrent collaterals of the ventral root fiber *m*: arborizations of the thin axon arising from sensory cells in the dorsal horn also
contribute to these plexuses.
B: The actual relationship between dorsal and ventral roots. *s*: unipolar spinal
ganglion cell; *m*: ventral root fiber. After coursing through the dorsal root, the
centripetal fiber of ganglion cell *s* reaches the dorsal funiculus, where it
bifurcates into ascending and descending branches that give rise to fine,
transverse collaterals, which surround motor cells in the ventral horn with
terminal arborizations. Individual dorsal root fibers give rise to several bifurcating collaterals of this kind.

white matter have a more delicate appearance. When the fibers in the white matter are examined in such material, it is clear that they are actually longitudinally directed nerve fibers separated by a large number of neuroglial processes.

Nerve fibers are, in fact, the axons of cells in the gray matter that run transversely toward the periphery before coursing longitudinally for a variable distance and then reentering the horns of the spinal gray matter.

A majority of these axons end by way of extensive, varicose, freely ending arborizations within the gray matter, where they share intimate contacts with nerve cells. Thus, the axons in the white matter are in fact longitudinal, arciform commissures that stretch between two or more levels of the gray matter, an arrangement that earlier anatomists had guessed but remained to be demonstrated in recent studies by Golgi and myself.

Collaterals of the White Matter   These structures were mentioned and described briefly by Golgi in 1880, and then forgotten entirely for about ten years until I studied them in detail in 1889. The existence of such fibers was then finally accepted by the scientific community, a step representing, in my opinion, the most important advance in our understanding of the texture of the spinal cord in thirty years. The most recent studies of Koelliker, van Gehuchten, Cl. Sala, von Lenhossék, and Retzius have confirmed the existence of these fibers and have provided additional information about their organization.

The collaterals are thin fibers that arise at right angles from axons in the funiculi of the spinal cord. They course transversely and converge upon the gray matter, where they give rise to freely ending, varicose terminal arborizations that vary in length.

The final branches of this arborization usually follow a winding course, give rise at right angles to small sprouts, and end in a nodule.

These collaterals may be studied easily in the embryonic chick spinal cord from the fifth day of incubation, when they appear as small buds on axons in the funiculi, to the sixteenth day, when they are fully developed and give rise to an exceedingly complex plexus throughout the entire thickness of the gray matter.

The behavior of collaterals arising in the different funiculi of the white matter varies somewhat.

A. Collaterals from the Ventral Funiculus (figure 3, H)   Such collaterals are the thickest, and arise from large axons in the funiculus. They course somewhat dorsally in irregular bundles, and ramify throughout the entire ventral horn, particularly around motor cells. As I suggested and as Koelliker described in detail, some of these collaterals reach the midline of the spinal cord and ramify in the ventral horn on the opposite side, thus forming the ventral collateral commissure (figure 3, I), which generally lies dorsal to the *ventral axonal commissure.*

B. Collaterals from the Lateral Funiculus   These collaterals course medially and tend to ramify in intermediate regions of the gray matter. A group of these collaterals reaches the dorsal commissure, where it forms one component of what I have called the gray commissure. The collateral fibers that cross the midline tend to form two bundles, one ventral and one middle, and end in the dorsal horn and central gray on the opposite side (figure 3, E and F).

C. Collaterals from the Dorsal Funiculus   The vast majority of these fibers arise from the dorsal roots, which also provide most of the fibers in the gracile (Goll) and cuneate (Burdach) fasciculi and in the marginal zone (Lissauer). Four groups of collaterals should be distinguished.

1. Sensory-Motor Collaterals (Koelliker's *reflexo-motor collaterals*) (figure 3, G)   These collaterals arise along the longitudinal course of dorsal root fibers, as well as occasionally from the parent axon itself before it bifurcates into ascending and descending branches; they end throughout the area of the ventral horn.

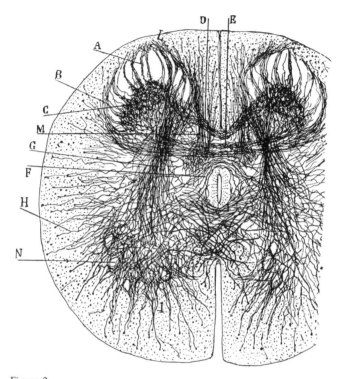

Figure 3
Transverse section through the rostral spinal cord of a newborn dog to show
the general arrangement of collaterals arising from fibers in the funiculi.
A: bundles of collaterals from the dorsal funiculus that course through the
substantia gelatinosa of Rolando; B: lateral collaterals following an arching
course; C: very thick plexus in the head of the dorsal horn that is formed by
the arborizations of collaterals from fibers in the dorsal funiculus; D: dorsal
arciform bundle of the gray commissure; E: middle bundle of the gray commissure; F: ventral arciform bundle; G: large sensory-motor bundle, most
probably arising from the dorsal roots (as collateral branches of the incoming
bifurcated root fibers); M: small fiber bundle destined for Clarke's column; H:
collateral bundles of the ventral funiculus; N: spaces occupied by motor cells
that are surrounded by the innumerable arborizations of collateral fibers; L:
the region giving rise to a great many of the fibers in the sensory-motor
bundle; I: collateral bundles of the ventral funiculus.

I shall consider these fibers in detail below because of their immense physiological importance as the major pathway underlying reflex movements.

2. Collaterals Destined for the Dorsal Horn (figure 3, A)   These collaterals are also quite numerous. They course through the substantia gelatinosa of Rolando in arching bundles and generate an extremely dense and tangled plexus in the head of the dorsal horn, forming the ventral border of the substantia gelatinosa (figure 3, C).

3. Collaterals to Clarke's Column (figure 3, M)   A small dorsoventrally oriented bundle that arises in the gracile fasciculus and ends entirely within Clarke's column as thick pericellular plexuses can be observed in newborn mammals and in avian embryos from the twelfth to the sixteenth day of incubation.

4. Collaterals Entering the Dorsal Commissure (figure 3, D)   A small bundle that arches ventrally arises primarily in the gracile fasciculus and courses through the dorsalmost part of the gray commissure to end in the head of the dorsal horn. The result of this arrangement is that the gray commissure is formed by three bundles of collaterals: a small ventral bundle arising from the ventral part of the lateral funiculus; a small middle bundle arising from the most distant parts of the lateral funiculus; and a small dorsal bundle that arises from the dorsal funiculus.

In summary, all of the funiculi give rise to two classes of collaterals. The terminal arborizations of some end in the gray matter on the same side, and the others (commissural) ramify in the gray matter on the opposite side.

Gray Matter
Leaving aside neuroglia, the gray matter consists of: (1) nerve cells and their dendrites; (2) the axons that these cells send to the white matter; (3) the ramifications of collaterals from the white matter; (4) the terminal arborizations of axons arising in the white matter or entering from the dorsal roots; and (5) the collaterals of certain axons that cross the gray matter on their way to the white matter. Together these components form an

exceedingly thick plexus that would be impossible to study analytically without the singular property of silver chromate to stain only a few types of fibers and cells in the gray matter of a particular section.

The morphological features of nerve cells are only slightly different in each horn of the spinal cord, except in the substantia gelatinosa of Rolando, which contains several unique cell types. Thus, the distinction between ventral and dorsal horns has more topographical than histological significance. The one feature that serves to distinguish different cell types is the behavior of their axons.

Based on this criterion, I have distinguished the five cell types illustrated in figure 4: (1) root cells, (2) commissural cells, (3) funicular cells, (4) multifunicular cells, and (5) short-axoned cells. Whereas the axon of the fifth type is confined to the gray matter, the other four cell types send their axon into the white matter, and are thus cells with long axons (Golgi motor cells).

1. Root Cells (figure 4, *k*)   These giant cells, the largest in the spinal cord, are found in the ventrolateral part of the ventral horn. They have a thick axon that usually lacks collaterals and crosses radially through the ventrolateral funiculus to enter the nearest motor root.

The dendrites of these cells are thick and highly branched, and can be divided into ventrolateral, dorsal, and medial groups. The medial dendrites bifurcate in the gray matter near the ventral commissure. Some of the branches reach the midline and enter the ventral horn on the other side after passing by similar dendrites from the other side (my dendritic commissure has also been observed by van Gehuchten and Sala). The ventrolateral processes end within the interstices of the ventrolateral funiculus, while the dorsal processes end in various parts of the dorsal horn.

2. Commissural Cells (figure 4, *m*)   These cells are smaller and have fewer dendrites than the root cells. Golgi had earlier demonstrated that they are found throughout the thickness of

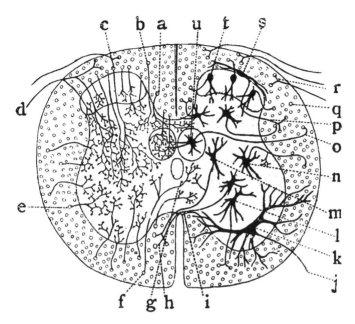

Figure 4
A diagrammatic representation of a section through the spinal cord showing relationships between its various components based on recent discoveries.
a: collaterals of the gracile fasciculus that form most of the dorsal commissure; *b*: collaterals from the same fasciculus that course to the dorsal horn; *c*: collaterals of the dorsal funiculus that reach the central gray and may extend to the ventral horn; *d*: a root fiber and its collaterals; *e*: collaterals of the ventral funiculus; *f*: collaterals that contribute to the formation of the ventral commissure; *g*: their course through the commissure; *h*: axon from a commissural cell that enters the ventral funiculus after passing through the ventral commissure; *i*: course of this axon in the commissure; *j*: axon from a large motor cell *k* that courses directly to the ventral root; *l*: a ventral funicular cell with its bifurcated axon; *m*: cell with a commissural axon; *n*: cell with an axon that gives rise to collaterals that form local connections; *o*: axon of a cell in Clarke's column; *p*: axon of cell *s*; *q*: axon cut transversely; *r*: bifurcation of a dorsal root fiber into ascending and descending branches; *s*: marginal cell of the substantia gelatinosa; *t*: small cell in the same region; *u*: cell body in Clarke's column.

the gray matter and that their axon crosses the midline ventrally (in the white commissure), continuing longitudinally in the ventrolateral funiculus of the opposite side.

I subsequently demonstrated that this is usually not a simple extension but rather involves a T-shaped division. This implies that the commissural axon divides and gives rise to an ascending and a descending branch when it reaches the white matter on the opposite side, a feature that was also observed by Koelliker and van Gehuchten.

3. Funicular Cells   I have applied this name to the many medium-sized cells throughout the gray matter that give rise to a longitudinal axon in the white matter on the same side of the spinal cord. The largest group of such cells, which lies in the ventral horn, sends its axons into the ventrolateral funiculus (figure 4, *n*), whereas cells in the dorsal horn send their axon to the dorsalmost part of the lateral funiculus. On the other hand, some cells in the substantia gelatinosa and the medial part of the dorsal horn send their functional process into the dorsal funiculus. Some of my observations also indicate that two cell types can be distinguished in Clarke's column: commissural cells with an axon that enters the ventral commissure, and lateral funicular cells with an axon that enters the lateral funiculus and joins the so-called cerebellar pathway (figure 4, *u*, *o*). Finally, it is worth pointing out that these fibers join the myelinated axons of the white matter in two ways. They either bend to continue as a single ascending or descending conductor, or they undergo a T-shaped division that gives rise to two conductors or longitudinal branches, one ascending and the other descending.

4. Multifunicular Cells   This term has been used to avoid periphrasis in referring to certain cells (which I was the first to observe) whose axon divides two or three times in the gray matter before entering two or three different regions of the white matter. For example, some cells give rise to an axon with one branch that enters the ventral funiculus on the same side and another branch that is destined for the ventral funiculus on the opposite side. Other cells give rise to an axon that divides into a fiber entering the dorsal funiculus and another fiber entering the lateral or ventral funiculus, and so on.

5. Short-Axoned Cells Golgi noted, and I confirmed, that there are neurons in the substantia gelatinosa of Rolando whose thin, flexuous axon gives rise to a freely ending terminal arborization that is restricted to the gray matter. These arborizations appear to interrelate different layers of neurons in the longitudinal dimension.

Substantia Gelatinosa of Rolando
This region of the dorsal horn contains many funicular cells as well as many so-called Golgi sensory or short-axoned cells. I have not as yet observed commissural cells in this region. Small bundles of collaterals from the dorsal funiculus, as well as many neuroglial filaments, pass between these cells.

From a morphological point of view, the substantia gelatinosa contains three types of neural elements that are arranged in three concentric zones: (1) horizontal or border cells; (2) piriform or fusiform cells, and (3) stellate or irregular cells.

The border cells are large, fusiform or triangular in shape, and lie between the substantia gelatinosa and dorsal funiculus, where they form an irregular series of neural elements. The polar dendrites follow the ventral border of the dorsal funiculus, where they ramify. The axon arises either from the lateral part of the cell body or from a dendrite and runs transversely to the dorsal part of the lateral funiculus, where it continues with a myelin sheath. In the initial part of its course, the axon runs ventrally through the substantia gelatinosa, where it may issue a few collaterals, and then turns to run laterally (figure 4, *s,p*).

The fusiform nerve cells are the smallest components of the spinal cord. They have a characteristic dorsoventral orientation with many sinuous, spiny, highly tangled dendrites, most of which arise from a ventral stem that stretches as far as the head of the dorsal horn. While the shape of these cells is quite variable, they are most commonly fusiform or piriform with the cell body lying dorsally. The axon often arises from the dorsal part of the cell body and courses either dorsally, laterally, or medially to contribute one or more fibers to the dorsal funiculus (figure 4, *t*).

The stellate cells lie nearest to the head of the dorsal horn and their many spiny dendrites fill the substantia gelatinosa and adjacent parts of the dorsal horn. The axon of some of these cells is directed longitudinally, like that of the Golgi sensory cells, and appears to end within the substantia gelatinosa itself. The axon of certain other cells courses medially to run in the cuneate fasciculus, while still others, which are quite small, course laterally to enter the dorsalmost part of the lateral funiculus, or Lissauer's marginal zone. I have even observed stellate cells with two axons in the pigeon embryo; one of these processes is directed to the inner, and the other to the outer, part of the dorsal funiculus. It is not clear whether this unusual arrangement persists in the adult, or whether it represents a stage in the embryonic development of the axon. It may, in fact, resemble the development of spinal ganglion cells and cerebellar granule cells, where the two axons merely represent two parts of a single functional process that arises from the cell body at a later stage. This appears to be the most likely explanation since it is not uncommon to find cells in the substantia gelatinosa that give rise to a multifunicular axon, that is, an axon that divides and supplies branches to two distinct parts of the dorsal funiculus, or to two different funiculi altogether.

Dorsal Roots
It is clear that fibers in the dorsal (sensory) roots arise from unipolar cells in the spinal ganglia. Several years ago Ranvier demonstrated that the single process arising from these cells bifurcates, with one branch coursing medially as a nerve fiber

in the dorsal root and the other branch coursing toward the periphery as a sensory fiber in the corresponding spinal nerve.

The disposition of the dorsal roots within the spinal cord has been one of the most difficult and controversial topics in anatomy, and hypotheses about the origin of these nerve fibers have already been mentioned. Thus, except for a group of root fibers that enters the dorsal funiculus and ascends through the white matter at least as far as the medulla, almost all of the dorsal root fibers disappear within a neural plexus that consists either of anastomosing dendrites (according to Gerlach and most other scientists) or of anastomosing axon collaterals and terminals (according to Golgi, Nansen, and others).

Despite these differences of opinion, there has been unanimous agreement on one point: each sensory axon remains separate in the white matter, whereas its branches ramify and anastomose in the gray matter.

This notion is completely erroneous. By 1887, Nansen had demonstrated that dorsal root fibers in glutinous mixine, the lowest species of fish, bifurcate in the white matter, with the branches coursing longitudinally and giving rise to collaterals that enter the gray matter. However, while many scientists accepted the validity of this observation, no one dared believe that this was a common feature of vertebrates, let alone mammals. Therefore, I was both surprised and skeptical when my initial studies of the spinal cord in birds and mammals revealed the presence of bifurcated dorsal root fibers with collaterals. These feelings were well founded; if my assertions were correct, they would cast serious doubt on the recent, very detailed studies of Bechterew, von Lenhossék, Obersteiner, Edinger, and others. Axons with a descending branch were not mentioned in any of these studies. On the other hand, the direct entry of sensory fibers into the substantia gelatinosa and the dorsal horn was established, and it had been shown that these fibers are collaterals or branches arising from either the principal stem or from the ascending and descending branches.

The results of these studies are valid, with the provision that a majority of the myelinated fibers described in the gray matter are collaterals from the dorsal columns or from the proximal part of a longitudinal branch of the dorsal root fibers. In fact, it should be pointed out that the vast majority of thin myelinated axons crossing the gray matter of the adult spinal cord are not direct extensions of dorsal root fibers but are instead collaterals arising in the white matter, for only the terminal arborizations of these collaterals lack myelin.

I continued to doubt these conclusions until a meeting of the German Anatomical Society in 1889, where my preparations convinced even the most reluctant observers. Since then my descriptions have been confirmed by Koelliker, van Gehuchten, Retzius, and even von Lenhossék, who treated them initially with the utmost caution.

Each dorsal root consists of centrifugal fibers and centripetal or sensory fibers.

The vast majority are centrifugal fibers, which can be divided into two bundles: the outer bundle contains thin fibers, while the inner bundle contains thick fibers, a distinction recognized by Bechterew, von Lenhossék, Edinger, Kahler, and others in material prepared with the Weigert-Pal method. These fibers arise from spinal ganglion cells and reach the dorsal funiculus, where they turn obliquely and bifurcate, giving rise to longitudinal ascending and descending branches. These branches appear to course several centimeters through the white matter before entering the gray matter, where they give rise to freely ending arborizations between components of the dorsal horn (figure 2, B, and figure 5, A) and substantia gelatinosa.

The results of recent unpublished studies have convinced me that the outer and inner bundles of centripetal fibers in 12- to 16-day-old chick embryos behave differently. The thin fibers in the outer bundle give rise to their final bifurcation in Lissauer's marginal zone and adjacent parts of the lateral funiculus. The branches issue very few collaterals, which are quite delicate and appear to end entirely within the dorsal horn.

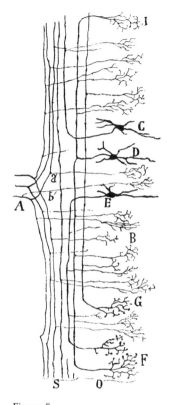

Figure 5

A semidiagrammatic longitudinal section through the dorsal funiculus, parallel to the entrance of the dorsal roots.

A: dorsal root; S: white matter; O: gray matter; C: dorsal funicular cell with a bending axon; D: another dorsal funicular cell whose axon bifurcates into ascending and descending branches; E: another cell with a bending axon that descends; F and G: the terminal arborizations of axons; B: the terminal arborizations of collaterals from the white matter; a': a collateral from the branch of a dorsal root fiber; b': a collateral from the stem of the same dorsal root fiber.

The inner bundle enters the dorsal columns where the thick fibers bifurcate for the last time. This bundle is the only source of large collaterals in the sensory-motor bundle.

When a dorsal root-stem fiber bifurcates, the branches leave at right angles, as do the thin collaterals of the branches, which enter the gray matter and give rise to elegant arborizations that are varicose and end freely near cell bodies in the dorsal and ventral horns.

As mentioned above, many dorsal root collaterals converge to form a dorsoventrally oriented bundle that traverses the dorsal horn and then fans out to arborize around motor cells throughout the ventral horn. This group of fibers, which I have called the sensory-motor (and Koelliker called the reflexo-motor) bundle, is quite important because it allows the sensory roots to communicate with the motor roots. The cell bodies and dendrites of motor cells receive sensory currents from collaterals in this bundle and reflect them through the ventral roots to the muscles. Reflex actions are thus explained more easily by the theory of action through contact or contiguity than by the plexus hypothesis, as illustrated recently in diagrams presented by Koelliker and Waldeyer. The contact theory also explains why weak sensory impressions produce limited muscle reflexes whereas stronger impressions evoke larger, more complex reflexes. In fact, weak sensory currents flow only through the initial collaterals of the root fiber to influence a small number of motor cells, whereas stronger sensory currents are transmitted throughout the length of the ascending and descending branches, as well as their collaterals and terminals, which contact and set into action vast numbers of motor cells (figure 2, B and figure 5 and 6).

It is also worth pointing out that the sensory current divides into two secondary currents that flow into the ascending and descending branches of the dorsal root fiber; thus, the flow of sensory currents is not necessarily centripetal as had been thought previously.

The problem of how sensory impressions reach the sensorium is still cloaked in mystery. However, the ascending and

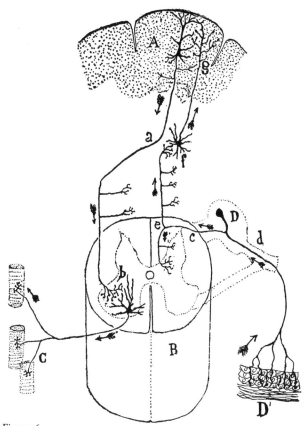

Figure 6

Diagram showing the course of voluntary motor impulses and conscious sensory impressions.

A: psychomotor region of the cerebral cortex; B: spinal cord; C: muscle fiber; D: spinal ganglion; D': skin.—The current associated with the motor impulse leaves a pyramidal cell in the psychomotor region of the brain, A, descends the length of the cell's axon, *a*, and passes through a terminal arborization at *b* to a spinal ventral horn cell, which then sends it along an axon to several muscle fibers C. The sensory current arises in the periphery, at D' for example, and passes through *d* to the spinal ganglion cell, D. The current continues along this cell's root fiber, *c*, which ascends through the dorsal funiculus, probably as far as the medulla, *f*. Here a new cell appears to carry the current all the way to the cerebral cortex, *g*, where its terminal arborizations contact and thus influence the dendrites of pyramidal cells. (Arrows indicate the direction of descending motor impulses on the left and ascending sensory impressions on the right.)

descending branches presumably give rise to terminal arborizations in the gray matter that may distribute currents in two ways. First, the collaterals and terminal arborizations may come in contact with cells in the dorsal horn, most of which give rise to an ascending axon in the lateral funiculus. And second, the collaterals may enter Clarke's column and make contact with cells whose axon ascends through the lateral funiculus in the cerebellar pathway.

Pyramidal Tracts

It is well known that the spinal cord contains two fiber bundles, the pyramidal tracts, that arise in the brain. The ventral bundle courses through the medialmost zone of the ventral funiculus, and is known as the direct pyramidal tract or Türck's bundle, while the dorsal bundle courses through the innermost part of the lateral funiculus. In certain preparations the arborizations of these fibers can be seen to end freely around cells (particularly root cells) in the ventral horn.

The pyramidal tracts conduct impulses for voluntary movement, although their terminal arborizations do not necessarily always contact the dendrites of ventral root (motor) cells.

The diagram in figure 6 shows the probable course taken by sensory impressions to the brain, as well as the course of the pyramidal tract, which transmits impulses related to voluntary movement to the ventral horn. This figure provides additional evidence that neural currents generated in the bosom of cortical pyramidal cells are *cellulipetal* in the dendrites and *cellulifugal* in the axon. Later in the book we shall argue strongly for the validity of this doctrine, which is confirmed in other parts of the nervous system and serves as a powerful tool for interpreting the direction of current flow in every cell of the various nerve centers.

The Spinal Cord of Lower Vertebrates

The work of Nansen, Retzius, and von Lenhossék in fish, of P. Ramón, Lawdowsky, Cl. Sala, and Sclavunos in amphibi-

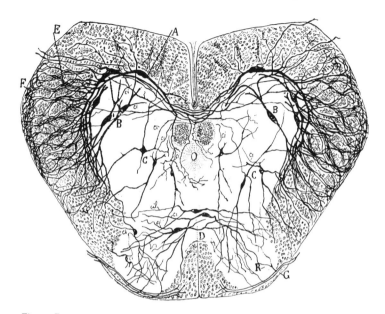

Figure 7

A transverse section through the spinal cord of *Lacerta agilis*.

A: motor cells of the ventral horn with medial processes that form the ventral dendritic commissure; B: commissural cells; C: funicular cells; D: dorsal dendritic commissure; E: various dendritic bundles that consist of dendrites from ventral root cells (A), funicular cells, and commissural cells (B). Together these bundles form the perimedullary plexus, F, which lies just deep to the pia mater at the level of the lateral, but not the dorsal, funiculus. Certain peripheral collaterals of the white matter, and perhaps certain nerve fiber terminals, join the perimedullary plexus; G: dorsal root; R: collateral of a sensory root fiber; *ci*: axons.

ans, and my own work in reptiles demonstrates that the structural plan of the spinal cord is identical in all vertebrates. Differences are related to the relative size of various bundles and to the extent of dendritic arborizations (figure 7).

Thus, the dendritic commissure is larger in the spinal cord of amphibians and reptiles; the outer dendrites of the ventral root and funicular cells contribute to the various bundles that form a perimedullary dendritic plexus just below the pia mater after crossing the white matter. More precisely, this plexus is centered in the lateral funiculus and does not extend into the dorsal funiculus. The results of my own studies, as well as those of Cl. Sala, indicate that certain peripheral collaterals of the white matter, as well perhaps as certain nerve fiber terminals, reach this plexus.

There is no perimedullary plexus in birds and mammals, or if there is, I have never been able to demonstrate it. On the other hand, dendritic bundles are still found in the white matter of birds and mammals, and it should come as no surprise that the latest studies have shown the presence of terminal arborizations arising from interstitial collaterals in the region of these bundles. Thus, fibers in the white matter give rise to collaterals that end locally without reaching the gray matter.

One other unusual feature of the reptilian and amphibian spinal cord is worth noting. The smallest dendrites are so thin and smooth that in certain instances they can readily be confused with the terminal parts of axons. This feature explains why Lawdowsky erroneously identified as axons some of the dendrites in the amphibian perimedullary plexus.

Chapter 2
The Cerebellum

No part of the nervous system is more appropriate than the cortical gray matter of the cerebellum for clarifying important questions about the shape and contacts of ganglion (nerve) cells. Unique features presented by the cerebellum include clearly differentiated cell layers, short axons, and dendritic arborizations that are perfectly aligned in a reproducible pattern.

Three concentric layers may be observed in a transverse section through a cerebellar folium. The first, or superficial, layer consists of grayish tissue that is referred to as the *molecular layer*. The second layer may be gray, yellowish, or reddish and is referred to as the *granular layer*. The third, or deep, layer lies in the center of each folium and is called the *white matter zone*.

Little was known about the structure of these layers before the application of recent methods. The molecular zone was considered a grainy mass containing scattered small nerve cells, although their shapes were not known. Vast numbers of small cells were known to lie in the granular zone, although again their nature was unclear. Finally, large oval cells between these two layers were known; it had been shown that their dendrites entered, and then somehow became lost, within the molecular layer, whereas their axon descended into the white matter. Golgi made important contributions to this field with his invaluable method, although he could not resolve the problem of intercellular connections. Because he failed to describe the course and termination of most types of nerve fibers, I have published the results of my own studies, the most interesting parts of which will now be summarized.

The Molecular or Granular Zone
This zone contains two cell types: Purkinje cells and small stellate cells.

Purkinje Cells   These cells can be observed in appropriate preparations, such as those described by Golgi (figure 8, *a*). The apical part of the cell body gives rise to one or more trunks that enter the molecular zone, where they expand into a luxuriant, flattened arborization that extends all the way to the surface of the cerebellum. Each branch of this arborization ends freely, and is studded with innumerable collateral spines that emerge at right angles. I was the first to observe these spines, which have recently been confirmed by van Gehuchten and Retzius.

The most interesting feature displayed by the arborizations of these cells is that they are flat and are arranged in a perfectly transverse orientation. Thus, if a folium is cut longitudinally, all of the Purkinje cells and their arborizations are displayed in profile, as shown earlier by Henle and Obersteiner.

The Purkinje cell axon acquires a myelin sheath near its origin and descends into the white matter. At the level of the second or third node of Ranvier, the axon gives rise to several ascending collaterals that ramify in the deep part of the molecular layer, where the arborizations assume a predominantly longitudinal orientation. These fibers make contact with the branches of different Purkinje cells a number of times, and may well serve to provide a measure of coordinated activity between these cells (figure 8, *o*).

Small Stellate Cells   These small cells are oriented in the transverse plane. The fact that they are neurons was recognized by Golgi, who identified the axon and showed that it runs horizontally and gives rise to ascending and descending collaterals.

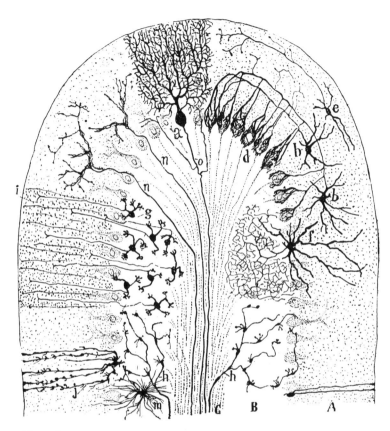

Figure 8
Semidiagrammatic transverse section through a mammalian cerebellar folium.
A: molecular zone; B: granular zone; C: white matter; *a:* Purkinje cell, front
view; *b:* small stellate cells of the molecular zone; *d:* descending terminal
arborizations that surround Purkinje cells; *e:* superficial stellate cells; *f:* large
stellate cells of the granular zone; *g:* granule cells with their long ascending
axons that bifurcate at *i; h:* mossy fibers; *i:* neuroglial cell with its plume; *m:*
neuroglial cell of the granular zone; *n:* climbing fibers; *o:* ascending collateral
of a Purkinje cell axon.

However, Golgi believed that an interstitial neural plexus provides the basis for intercellular communication and was unable to determine where these axons terminate.

I had the pleasure of resolving this issue after extensive work in the cerebellum of birds (1888) and then of mammals. The results were stunning. They established for the first time how axons terminate in nerve centers. Previously, nerve fibers had been traced for some distance through the gray matter, but no one had observed their mode of termination. It is easy to appreciate the satisfaction and emotion I felt in publishing this discovery in view of my suspicion that it was not an isolated fact but rather the foundation of a law that governs the relationship between all nerve cells. I am convinced by virtually all of my recent studies that the impression of having found the key to understanding central neural connections was not idle speculation; they have confirmed and extended a fundamental relationship throughout the nervous system.

First, I recognized that typical deep stellate cells give rise to a very long, curving axon that not only runs parallel to the surface of the cerebellum (as described by Golgi and Fusari), but also maintains a strictly transverse orientation, parallel to the plane of the Purkinje cell dendrites. However, the most important point is that all of the descending collaterals and terminal arborizations of the stellate cell axon ramify to produce a thick plexus that is intimately related to the Purkinje cell bodies. Thus, each Purkinje cell body is, in a way, surrounded by a kind of basket formed by an extremely dense, varicose terminal arborization (figure 8, d). These unique arborizations were called *Endkörben* (terminal baskets) by Koelliker in a study that confirmed our own work. The group of fibers that surrounds a Purkinje cell condenses around the basal part of the cell body to form a kind of brush point that envelopes the initial part of its axon, which is not myelinated. Based on this short description and figure 8, d, it is clear that this arrangement allows a dynamic relationship—a true point of current transmission—to be established between stellate and Purkinje cells.

The Granular Layer

Granule Cells   These very small cells, which form a dense mass deep to the molecular zone, are four to six microns in diameter and have very little cytoplasm. Golgi demonstrated several different processes arising from these elements and presumed that they were nerve cells. However, he did not clarify how the dendrites end, and could not follow the axon.

These cells have three or four short *dendrites*, all of which end in a fingerlike arborization that appears to surround or touch the cell body of neighboring granule cells.

The *axon* is very thin and climbs toward the molecular zone where it divides in a T to give rise to a longitudinal fiber. These fibers, which divide at different levels in the molecular zone, run parallel to the length of a folium, and thus perpendicular to the Purkinje cell dendrites. These parallel fibers do not issue collaterals, and extend the length of a folium before ending freely as a swelling near the white matter. We may conclude from this that the parallel fiber, which arises from the bifurcation of a granule cell axon, presents the simplest example of an axon terminal (figure 9, *b*).

Given the enormous length of a folium in the adult mammalian cerebellum, it is clearly not possible to follow the entire course of a parallel fiber. Fortunately, however, this is not the case in lower vertebrates such as reptiles and amphibians, or in the fetus of small mammals, where it is relatively easy to examine the parallel fiber in great detail. It is also worth mentioning in passing that the arrangement of the granule cells and their axon, as well as the Purkinje cells and the white matter, is essentially the same in all vertebrates, as demonstrated by my brother, and more recently by Falcone and Schaper.

If we pause to consider that innumerable parallel fibers contact the spines of Purkinje cell dendrites, and recall that no other components of the molecular layer interact with parallel fibers, at least in a direct or effective way, we come naturally

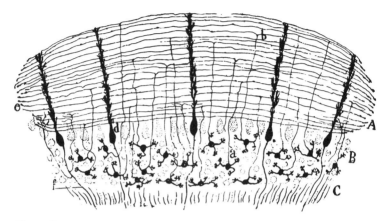

Figure 9
Semidiagrammatic longitudinal section through a cerebellar folium.
A: molecular zone; B: granular zone; C: white matter; *a:* ascending axon of a
granule cell; *b:* bifurcation of this axon and the formation of a parallel fiber;
d: Purkinje cell as seen in profile; *c:* terminal swelling of a parallel fiber; *f:*
Purkinje cell axon.

to the spirit of the hypothesis that these fibers establish a
contact point between granule cells and Purkinje cells.

An equally interesting consequence of this histological organization is that the parallel fiber of a granule cell can probably influence all of the Purkinje cells along its beam, which
stretches the length of a folium. Conversely, because current
flows in both directions, each Purkinje cell in a particular
longitudinal zone of a folium can receive influences from all
of the granule cells in the subjacent part of the folium.

Large Stellate Cells   A few large cells that have been described
quite well by Golgi are also found in the granular zone. Their
dendrites radiate in all directions, even extending through
wide regions of the molecular zone. Shortly beyond its origin,
the tortuous axon dissolves into innumerable branches that
disappear among the granule cells. Golgi held that this arborization joins a dense plexus that includes all of the nerve fibers

in the cerebellum. In my opinion, however, terminals arising from the stellate cell axon end freely as arciform varicosities on granule cell bodies (figure 8, *f*).

White Matter
The white matter contains three types of nerve fibers: (1) the descending axons of Purkinje cells; (2) thick, ascending fibers that ramify among the granule cells (mossy fibers); and (3) thick, ascending fibers that ramify in the molecular layer (climbing fibers).

Descending Axons   These axons, which are rather sparse, have already been described above. They descend from Purkinje cells and converge in the white matter before leaving the cerebellum to end in other nerve centers.

Mossy Fibers   I so named these thick, richly arborized fibers because the characteristic knotty thickenings (bristling with short, diverging processes that form rosettes) that are displayed along their length resemble moss covering a tree. These swellings were confirmed by Koelliker, although he was unsure of their significance and was thus inclined to regard them as artifacts. It is now clear, however, that they are a normal, characteristic feature (figure 8, *h*) in view of the fact that they have been described and drawn by van Gehuchten, von Lenhossék, and Retzius, and their existence in fish, amphibians, and reptiles was confirmed by my brother.

These fibers and their branches do not extend beyond the granular layer, where they end freely in a nodule, or in the center of ascending rosettes analogous to those just described. These branches appear to come in contact with granule cells, relaying current to them from nerve centers that remain to be determined. Is it possible that these fibers constitute terminals of the spinal projection to the cerebellum?

Climbing Fibers   These thick, myelinated fibers branch very infrequently as they course through the granule cells. However, once they reach the molecular zone they wrap around the ascending trunk of the Purkinje cells like creepers along the branches of a tropical tree. They end by way of a varicose, plexiform arborization that touches the large primary and secondary dendrites of Purkinje cells. When stained selectively with silver chromate, the arborizations can be seen to reflect faithfully the outline of Purkinje cell dendrites.

This arrangement provides another elegant example of neural connections through contact, much like Rouget's muscle end plate. In both cases an axon ramifies on a giant cell, where it transmits excitation from another center.

Unfortunately, the nerve cells that give rise to climbing fibers have not yet been identified.

This brief summary of cerebellar structure, which has been confirmed by the recent work of Koelliker, von Lenhossék, His, Waldeyer, van Gehuchten, Retzius, and Falcone, leads to the following conclusions:

1. The function of dendrites and the cell body is to transmit neural currents in light of my observations that certain axons ramify and end freely on dendrites.

2. Different types of connections can be established with different parts of a nerve cell, and thus remain independent. For example, I have been able to show that each part of the cell body and dendrites of Purkinje cells is associated with a distinct type of axon terminal arborization. The cell body is surrounded by the terminal baskets of molecular layer stellate cells, the primary and secondary dendrites are related to inputs from the spinal cord or brain by way of the climbing arborizations, and the terminal dendritic branches are contacted by the axons of granule cells, the parallel fibers.

3. Dynamic connections between nerve cells appear to be mediated through contacts between axon terminals on the one hand, and the cell bodies and dendrites on the other. Different modes of communication cannot be excluded, but this is certainly the most general and important.

In short, these laws of intercellular relationships are equally valid in the spinal cord and other nerve centers.

Chapter 3
The Cerebral Cortex

Neurologists have shown a particular interest in carrying out research aimed at clarifying the structure of the mammalian cerebral cortex. Those deserving special mention for the understanding they have brought to this particularly difficult subject include Gerlach, Wagner, Schültze, Deiters, Stieda, Krause, Koelliker, Exner, Meynert, Edinger, Betz, Golgi, Martinotti, Fleschig, and Retzius.

Before Golgi's famous book (*Sulla fina anatomia degli organi centrali del sistema nervoso*) appeared in 1886, our knowledge about the structure of cortical gray matter could be summarized as follows.

1. The gray matter contains pyramidal cells with a branching dendrite that is oriented toward the surface of the brain, and a descending, unbranched axon. The presence of an axon had only been established for giant cells.

2. The gray matter is divided into a number of layers each containing distinctive elements. According to Meynert's description, which was blindly followed by Huguenin and many others, the following layers, from superficial to deep, could be identified. The first layer contains neuroglial cells, nerve fibers, and a few triangular or fusiform ganglion cells; the second layer contains small pyramidal cells; the third layer, or ammonic formation, consists of large pyramidal cells like those found in Ammon's horn; the fourth layer contains small triangular or spherical cells; and the fifth layer consists of fusiform cells.

Very little was known about the shape of the dendritic shaft and the larger processes of cells in the various layers, and there was complete ignorance about the arrangement of smaller dendrites and most parts of the axons. In fact, Gerlach's concept of the dendritic plexus, which was discussed above, was used to explain the dynamic relationship between cells in the cerebral cortex.

3. It was known that a large number of myelinated fibers converge in the deep zones to form small bundles, whereas they assume a more irregular and plexiform arrangement in the middle zones. The latter fibers were thought to continue superficially as the axons or basilar processes of pyramidal cells, while the deep fibers were thought to consist of nerve fibers associated with the corona radiata.

Such was the state of our knowledge about the microscopic structure of the cerebral cortex when Golgi arrived on the scene with his analytical method for staining nerve cells. His studies firmly established a number of points.

1. He discovered the complex branching pattern of pyramidal cell dendrites, and demonstrated that they do not anastomose.

2. He demonstrated that virtually all cortical pyramidal cells give rise to a descending axon with a number of branching collaterals.

3. He differentiated two classes of neurons in the gray matter, based on the properties of their axon. In one class, the axon ramifies extensively before ending locally, and in the other the axon gives rise to many collaterals but continues as a myelinated fiber into the white matter. Golgi followed my lead in attributing a sensory role to the former and considered the latter to have a motor function.

4. He demonstrated the correct structure of the neuroglia, attributing the entire connective framework of nerve centers to the intermingling (without anastomoses) of innumerable thin processes radiating from these cells (Deiters' cells) like a spider web.

Only a few tentative physiological correlates were proposed, such as a distinction between sensory and motor cells, which had already been raised, and Golgi's ideas were largely confirmed by Tartuferi, Mondino, Fusari, Nansen, Koelliker, Todlt and Kahler, Obersteiner, Edinger, Retzius, and myself.

Little has been added to our knowledge of cerebral morphology in the six years following the publication of this important work by Golgi. However, it is worth mentioning that during this period Fleschig (1890) did employ a special staining method to reveal the existence of myelinated collaterals in the cortex, and Martinotti (1891) demonstrated that certain pyramidal cells give rise to an axon that ascends to form one component of the fibers in the first layer.

Despite the authoritative research of so many workers and the introduction of new analytical methods, the problems associated with understanding the structure and function of the cerebral cortex remain numerous and transcend the immediate physical properties of the cortex.

What are the features of nerve cells in the first layer? Do the axon collaterals form a plexus or do they end freely like the collaterals arising from the white matter of the spinal cord? What cell type gives rise to the fibers in the corpus callosum? Are the cells that contribute to the association, projection, and commissural pathways found in distinct layers through the thickness of the cortex, or are they intermingled with other elements as they are in the spinal cord? Where does excitation begin in a pyramidal cell, and what is the significance of its characteristic plume, which is oriented toward the surface of the brain in all vertebrates? Does the law of intercellular connections through dendrosomatic contacts govern relationships in the cerebral cortex (as I have already shown to be the case in other parts of the brain, spinal cord, olfactory bulb, and so on)?

It is clear that over the last two decades anatomists and physiologists have offered rather ingenious solutions to many of these problems. However, they are based on incomplete observations or on anatomical and pathological observations that are open to alternative interpretations. It has therefore become necessary to reexamine all aspects of this problem with impartial application of the analytical methods that provided us with such excellent results in the spinal cord and cerebellum.

The organization of the cerebral cortex is perhaps the most difficult challenge faced by anatomy. The supreme dignity of the organ, together with the inextricable complexity of its underlying mechanisms, demands an immensely complex framework that only the wisest of scholars can begin to untangle, and within which even those who believe that nature can elaborate multiple, highly refined activities from simple mechanisms and schematic formulas become confused and lose their way again and again. It has also become clear that the approach used by Golgi and his students, based on an excellent method for revealing certain aspects of cellular morphology, is not the most appropriate for establishing the general organization of cortical connections. Almost all of the workers who have applied modern techniques to this problem have attacked the brain of humans and large mammals. However, because of the long distances involved, as well as the intricate and labyrinthine organization of the neural framework, it is virtually impossible to follow an axon or one of its collaterals from its origin to its site of termination in these brains.

On the other hand, in the embryo and newborn of small mammals such as mice, rats, bats, or guinea pigs the layers are thinner, the distances are shorter, and nerve fibers are stained more reliably. Under these conditions it is possible to determine with certainty the origin, course, and termination of at least some nerve fibers. I therefore developed this approach, whose advantages allowed me to discover several features that have at least slightly broadened our knowledge of the cortex. This new information has not provided answers to all of our questions about cortical organization (because of its complexity an insurmountable task), although it may lay the groundwork for the time when this enterprise is closer to being resolved.

The results of this work can be generalized reliably to the brains of humans and higher mammals since the brain is essentially identical in all mammals. The only differences are in microscopic form and in the relative volume of particular components used in its construction.

With this in mind, we shall now begin a detailed account of the cerebral cortex, devoting particular attention to structural arrangements that are common to all mammals and thus may be regarded as fundamental characteristics of cortical architecture.

It is possible to distinguish four layers in the cortex. The first is a molecular zone; the second is a layer of small pyramidal cells; the third is a layer of large pyramidal cells; and the fourth is a layer of polymorph cells. The first and fourth layers are rather well defined (limitrophic), whereas the second and third layers differ in so far as their borders are blurred by gradual transitions (figure 10).

Molecular Zone
This layer has a finely granular or reticulated appearance when examined in sections of the brain that have been stained with nothing more than carmine or aniline dyes. Scattered small nuclei of glial cells can be seen, particularly near the pia mater, along with a very small number of larger nuclei that are associated with a triangular or fusiform dendritic process and probably correspond to nerve cells.

Koelliker discovered a group of horizontal myelinated fibers in the most superficial part of the molecular zone; this was confirmed by Exner using his osmic acid-ammonia method, as well as by Edinger, Obersteiner, Todlt, Martinotti, and others using the Weigert-Pal method, which provided even better results (figure 13, A).

Little or nothing was known about the origin of these fibers, only a few of which descend toward the deeper layers of the cortex, until two years ago when Martinotti used the Golgi method to demonstrate two important facts. First, certain pyramidal cells give rise to an ascending axon that bends and assumes a horizontal course through the superficial part of the molecular zone. And second, the vast majority of horizontal

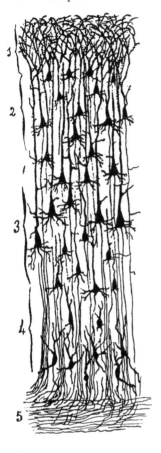

Figure 10
Transverse section through the gray matter of a cortical gyrus.
(1) molecular layer; (2) layer of small pyramidal cells; (3) layer of large pyramidal cells; (4) layer of polymorph cells; (5) white matter.

fibers in the molecular zone branch repeatedly like the terminal arborizations of axons.

Nevertheless, the origin of most of the horizontal nerve fibers in the molecular zone remains to be determined. Because the superficial layer contains endogenous beaded fibers that are much thicker and more numerous than those descending to deeper zones, I had come to suspect that perhaps all of the thick fibers, as well as many of the thinner fibers, arise from endogenous cells of the still poorly understood first layer, and that earlier researchers were inclined to consider them neuroglial cells because they were unable to stain them with the Golgi method.

These suspicions have been confirmed in my own work on young small animals, which revealed the presence of three distinct cell types.

1. Polygonal cells   These medium-sized cells (figure 11, D) give rise to between four and six dendrites that branch several times while coursing in various directions, including some that descend into the layer of small pyramidal cells. The axon is thin and usually arises from one side of the cell body or from a large dendrite. It courses obliquely or horizontally through the molecular zone and branches several times. The resulting collaterals are quite long and varicose, and follow a course

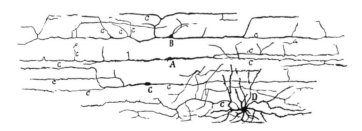

Figure 11
Special cells in the molecular layer of the cerebral cortex in a one-day-old dog.
A: fusiform cell; B: triangular or stellate cell; C: another fusiform cell; D: a polygonal cell with many dendrites and an axon that branches many times; *c:* axons.

parallel to the surface of the cortex. These axons never descend to the white matter, unlike those of pyramidal cells.

Special cells of the molecular zone   My latest studies have revealed the existence of two types of horizontal cells: 1) *fusiform cells* (figures 11, A and C) with two polar dendrites that bend somewhat in coursing toward the surface of the brain, and 2) *triangular or stellate cells* (figure 11, B) with horizontally oriented dendrites that issue ascending branches at right angles along their course. These two cell types have the peculiar feature of giving rise to two or more axons that stretch horizontally throughout the thickness of the molecular zone, where they divide several times at right angles and thus encompass a truly vast region.

Because I was unable to follow the entire course of the large branches that looked like dendrites, and because I suspected that these branches may assume the thin, smooth appearance and branching pattern of axons near their sites of termination, a new series of studies has been undertaken in the occipital region (corresponding to the band of Gennari or Vicq d'Azyr) of rabbits and guinea pigs. The molecular layer is quite thick in these species, and the cells of interest are remarkably abundant. These studies were difficult to carry out successfully for two reasons. First, other nerve cell processes are almost always stained in the molecular layer along with the cells of interest, thus creating a good deal of confusion. And second, the irregular course and enormous range (up to 0.7 mm) of the processes that look like dendrites often prevents their entire length to be observed within a single section.

Nevertheless, after many attempts I have succeeded in staining a number of these cells (see figure 11) and determining how the large processes arise from them. These processes course either horizontally or obliquely and gradually acquire the features of axons (figure 11, A), or give rise to two, three, or even more branches, each with the appearance of an axon.

In view of this, the special cells in the molecular layer of the cerebral cortex should be regarded as a class of nerve cells in which dendrites cannot be distinguished from axons, or better yet, in which all of the processes are equivalent to nerve fibers on the basis of morphological criteria.

Thus, my initial description should be modified in the following way:

2. Fusiform type   These oval or fusiform cells are oriented in the horizontal plane (figures 11, A and C) and give rise to two large polar trunks that are relatively straight. The edges of these trunks are rather smooth and give rise at right angles to several ascending branches that curve when they approach the surface of the brain and then branch again, giving rise to two or more quite long, varicose fibers that look like axons. These fibers ramify (almost always at right angles) entirely within the region of the molecular layer. Throughout their length, and particularly at bends (figure 11, C), the large trunks give rise to very thin, horizontally oriented branches that are quite long and in turn give rise to ascending collaterals. As shown in figure 11 A, it is not uncommon to observe a polar trunk that becomes gradually thinner without changing direction, and becomes transformed into a single or double axon.

3. Triangular or stellate type (figure 11, B)   The perikarya of this cell type give rise to three or more trunks, a feature that distinguishes it from the previous type with two polar shafts. Despite their initial course, the trunks of the triangular or stellate cells quickly assume a horizontal course and travel quite some distance, gradually transforming into small nerve fibers of the molecular zone.

There are many other varieties of this cell type, although the features displayed by their processes are similar.

These special cells are found in the molecular layer throughout all parts of the cortex. However, it seems clear from studies in the ventral occipital region of the rabbit that they usually lie in the deep or inner half of this layer, in contrast to the ordinary stellate cells (with a single axon) that are concentrated in the outer half of the layer.

Analogous or very similar cells are also found in larger mammals. I have occasionally stained cow and dog fetuses successfully, and here the processes, which are quite varicose, assume the appearance of embryonic nerve fibers at an early stage of development. I am convinced that these neural elements are also found in the human brain. The drawings that accompany Retzius' work on the cerebral cortex of the human fetus prove that he stained such cells, although not completely. In addition, Retzius now concedes that certain cells in the molecular layer that he originally believed were glial in nature probably correspond to the multipolar cells just described.

In summary, these elements constitute a specific cell type. However it is necessary to distinguish them from what might be considered an analogous cell type in the retina, the amacrine cell. These cells give rise to thin, radiating processes that are varicose, course horizontally, and have the features characteristic of nerve fibers. The most obvious difference between these amacrine cells and special cells of the cortex is that the latter give rise to pseudoaxonal branches that end on what are clearly dendrites, as well as on the trunks of the special cells themselves. However, it is worth pointing out that retinal amacrine cells and special cortical cells share one feature in common: both cell types are found entirely within molecular zones, that is, in regions containing the dendritic bouquets of underlying ganglion cells.

These unique cellular elements have been examined again in a recent study by Retzius (June 1893) of human and other mammalian embryos. He has confirmed my view that these special cells give rise to a number of processes that have features in common with nerve fibers. However, he also noted a feature that was rarely apparent in my preparations, namely that the ascending collaterals end in a large bulb at the very surface of the brain. Because these observations were made in the embryo, before development is complete, I am inclined to regard these submeningeal ascending branches as a developmental feature, much like those observed during the development of many other cell types, including cerebellar granule cells and bipolar spinal ganglion cells.

The gathering in the molecular layer of these many endogenous fibers, along with those ascending from the deeper layers, results in a very thick plexus of contact sites for the ascending terminal dendrites of pyramidal cells to pass through (figure 13, A). It is impossible to consider this unique arrangement, found throughout the vertebrate series, as anything other than a clear example of neural transmission *through contact*, or *contiguity*, much like that taking place in the cerebellum between parallel fibers and the dendritic tree of Purkinje cells. Such contacts in the molecular zone of the cerebral cortex also occur in the transverse or oblique plane, since the terminal branches of pyramidal cells display short collateral spines in regions where the thinnest unmyelinated nerve fibers are concentrated.

Before examining the other cortical layers in detail, it is worth noting the general morphological features of different types of pyramidal cells, as well as the layers in which they are found.

General Morphological Characteristics of Pyramidal Cells
The soma of such cells is shaped like a cone or pyramid and the axon invariably arises from the base, which faces the deep part of the cortex. The cells have a large number of dendrites that can be divided into groups according to their site of origin: an ascending shaft or primary expansion, collaterals of the ascending shaft, and basal processes arising from the cell body (figures 10 and 12, D).

The shaft is quite thick and ascends toward the surface parallel to the shafts of other pyramidal cells. It spreads into a splendid tuft or bouquet of dendritic branches that ends freely among nerve fibers in the molecular zone. Taken together, these distal tufts form an extremely thick dendritic plexus, which gives to this part of the cortex its finely reticulated appearance in ordinary preparations stained with carmine.

According to Golgi and Martinotti, these dendrites come into contact with blood vessels or with neuroglial cells. How-

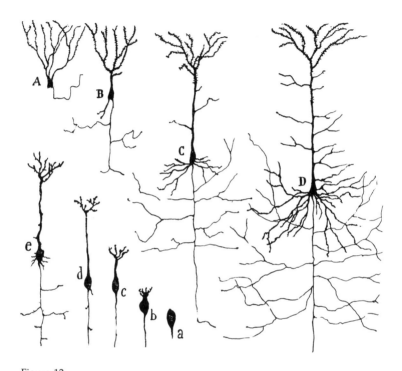

Figure 12
A diagram of pyramidal cell development in vertebrates.
The upper series of drawings illustrates the appearance of the psychic cell in
different vertebrates. A: frog; B: wall lizard; C: rat; D: human. The lower series
of drawings illustrates the developmental phases that psychic or pyramidal
cells pass through. *a:* a neuroblast without a dendritic shaft; *b:* appearance of
the shaft and terminal tuft; *c:* a more developed shaft; *d:* the appearance of
axon collaterals; *e:* the formation of dendrites from the cell body and the shaft.

ever, these branches do not in fact make this choice; they are distributed and end within the confines of the molecular zone, in the region of axon terminal arborizations, as Retzius has verified in the human fetus.[1]

I have referred to the dendritic shaft as primary because it is the first dendrite to appear during the development of this cell type, as illustrated in figure 12.

The lateral processes of the shaft arise at right or acute angles in association with a swelling and then course near the shaft, dividing several times and ending freely.

The basal processes arise from the pyramidal cell soma and course either horizontally or into the deeper layers, while branching several times and disappearing in neighboring regions. As noted above, *the axon* originates at the base of the pyramidal cell soma or from the origin of one of the basal dendrites. It descends through all layers of the cerebral cortex and enters the white matter, where it continues as a myelinated fiber. It had been thought that the descending axon always bends as it enters the white matter. However, I have demonstrated that the axons often bifurcate, thus giving rise to two myelinated fibers in the white matter. During its course through the gray matter the axon issues six to ten thin collaterals at right angles. These collaterals may course horizontally or obliquely, and end by way of two or three extremely delicate branches.

This is the basic form of the mammalian pyramidal cell, which we might also refer to as the *psychic cell,* bearing in mind its special morphology and restriction to the layers of the cerebral cortex, the substratum of the highest neural activity.

In descending the vertebrate ladder, the shape of the psychic cell becomes simpler, with its length and volume decreasing in parallel.

In amphibia (figure 12, A), the dendrites are condensed into a terminal bouquet that ramifies in the molecular zone, which

1. I have observed the same arrangement in the occipital region of the infant cortex—AZOULAY.

appears to be unusually well developed in these animals. Thus, *shaft* collaterals and basal processes are not found in amphibia.

In reptiles (figure 12, B) there is also a peripheral shaft, although it does not yet give rise to collaterals. The basal processes of mammals are represented by a descending process that originates in the cell body and branches to a limited extent.

Second Layer, or Zone of Small Pyramidal Cells
This zone contains many small to medium-sized (10 to 12 μ) polyhedral or pyramidal cells.

Since the general arrangement of the pyramidal cells that form the second layer of the cerebral cortex is well known, only a few additional features need to be pointed out (figure 10).

The size of these cells, along with the length of their peripheral shaft, increases according to their location from superficial to deep. The apical shaft often divides near the cell body and ends in an elaborate tuft or bouquet that is intermingled with those of other pyramidal cells throughout most of the thickness of the molecular layer. These cells also give rise to a number of ramified basal processes.

The axon of these cells is very thin, and as it descends it gives rise to four or five thin collaterals that branch once or twice at some distance from the point of origin. I have occasionally observed that the highest collaterals of these axons reach as far as the molecular zone itself (figure 13, *d*).

How do these collaterals end? Golgi, who discovered them, presumed that they branch repeatedly and then anastomose with other similar collaterals, thus participating in the formation of a continuous interstitial plexus in the gray matter.

This is one of the monumental problems that can only be solved by resorting to studies of ontogeny and comparative anatomy. Collaterals in the human and in larger mammals are extraordinarily long, and cannot be followed to their site of termination in any one section, no matter how thick.

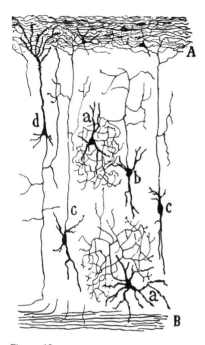

Figure 13
A section through the cortical gray matter of the brain.
A: molecular layer; B: white matter; *a:* cell with a short axon that arborizes extensively; *b:* cell with an ascending axon that does not reach the molecular layer; *c:* cells with an ascending axon that ramifies in the molecular layer; *d:* small pyramidal cell.

On the other hand, the collaterals in the embryos and newborn of small mammals are extremely short, where it is obvious that they end in a varicosity rather than an arborization. If young enough fetuses are used, the entire process of collateral growth can be observed from the moment they consist of nothing more than simple varicose processes arising from the axon, to the time they develop terminal branches (figure 12, d, e).

It is easy to confirm a similar arrangement in adult small mammals such as the rat, bat, and white mouse, although the distances involved are much greater than in embryos (figure 12, C).

The Third Layer. or Layer of Large Pyramidal Cells (Meynert's Ammonic Layer)

The only feature that distinguishes this layer from the one above it is the larger size of its cell bodies (20 to 30 μ), and the increased length and thickness of their peripheral shaft. Superficial parts of this layer blend with the second layer because the size of the cells gradually decreases, whereas deeper parts of the layer are more clearly defined. Nevertheless, large pyramidal cells are not infrequently observed in the middle of the polymorph zone (figure 10, 3).

The axons are very thick and descend with an almost straight trajectory to the white matter, where they generally continue as projection fibers. Some of the axons bifurcate upon reaching the white matter or give rise to a large collateral that appears destined for the corpus callosum (figure 16, B and G).

As they course through the gray matter these axons issue six to eight horizontal or oblique collaterals, each of which divides two or three times. The thinnest branches end freely in a varicosity.

The ascending shaft and basal processes are similar to those described for the small pyramidal cells.

Layer of Polymorph Cells (figure 10, 4; and figure 16, D)

Although this layer contains a few giant or medium-sized pyramidal cells with a peripheral shaft that ascends toward the molecular zone, most of the cells have an oval, fusiform, triangular, or polygonal shape, and have two characteristic features. First, although there are exceptions, the peripheral shafts are not rigorously oriented; second, they never reach the molecular zone to mix with the tufts or bouquets of all of the pyramidal cells. In fact, many of these cells lack a peripheral shaft, and instead give rise to two or more short, oblique processes. In addition, there are a number of cells with three thick dendrites, two of which extend to the white matter.

The axon is thin and descends, giving rise to three or four collaterals that branch several times. When the axon reaches the white matter, it either bends or undergoes a T-shaped division, continuing as one or two myelinated fibers.

Short-Axoned Cells (figure 13)   The three deep layers of cortex contain a small number of scattered neurons that fall into two classes and share the unusual feature that their axon ramifies and ends entirely within the thickness of the gray matter.

These two cell types include the sensory cells described by Golgi, and the cells with ascending axons described by Martinotti.

Golgi's sensory cells (figure 13, *a*) are typically polygonal in shape and issue dendrites in all directions. The axon arises from either the upper or lateral part of the cell body and may course in almost any direction for a short distance before breaking up into a freely ending arborization that surrounds the perikarya of neighboring cells.

Golgi, who discovered these cells, thought that they must play a role in sensory activity because the axon quickly loses its individuality. As I shall discuss below, the evidence taken as a whole does not support this conclusion. They are simply short-axoned cells that appear to provide a mechanism for interrelating neighboring cells without providing clues as to the nature of their function.

The cells with an ascending axon (figure 13, C) were first mentioned by Martinotti. Those of us who have studied them in small mammals find that they are scattered throughout the three deeper layers, although they are particularly common in the polymorph zone. They are either fusiform or triangular in shape, and have both ascending and descending dendrites. The axon, which may arise from the shaft of an ascending dendrite, climbs almost vertically to the molecular zone where it divides into two or three large branches that ramify horizontally and give rise to extremely thick terminal arborizations. I have occasionally observed that the terminal arborizations appear to ramify within the layer of small pyramidal cells rather than in the first layer (figure 13, *b*).

White Matter

The white matter contains four types of fibers: *projection fibers; callosal or commissural fibers; association fibers;* and *centripetal or terminal fibers.* All of these fibers appear to be intermingled in the white matter of the cerebral cortex of large mammals (dog, sheep, cow, human, etc.) in view of the fact that it is absolutely impossible to determine the origin or termination of individual fibers by direct observation. Fortunately, these analytical problems are less acute in small mammals, where it is more practical to trace these fibers over longer distances.

Projection fibers (figure 15, *a* and C)   All parts of the cortex give rise to such fibers, which converge in the corpus striatum and then enter the cerebral peduncles. In small mammals, these fibers issue a large collateral as they reach the top of the corpus callosum. The projection fibers then collect into small descending bundles, separated by regions of gray matter that receive a number of very thin collaterals from the bundles. There is also a group of projection axons that passes through the sheet of callosal fibers and the corpus striatum without issuing any collaterals at all.

Which cells give rise to the projection fibers? Some authors, including Monakow and others, have assumed that they arise exclusively from the giant pyramidal cells, in contrast to the association and callosal fibers that were thought to arise from the small pyramidal cells.

Although my own observations on this point are far from complete, they seem to establish beyond doubt that projection fibers arise from both large and small pyramidal cells, as well as from some of the polymorph cells. This mixture of cell sizes may explain why the small bundles of projection fibers descending through the corpus striatum contain a scattering of large axons.

It has not been possible to observe directly the final destination of these projection fibers in our anatomical material. However, results obtained in pathological material and with Fleschig's method have taught us that many such fibers contribute to the *pyramidal tract*, the descending pathway for voluntary motor impulses.

Association Fibers (figure 14)   These fibers probably arise in all three cell layers of the cerebral cortex (that is, from small and large pyramidal cells, and from polymorph cells), although no one but myself has been able to observe such fibers arising directly from polymorph cells and from a small number of

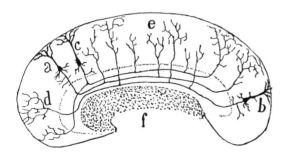

Figure 14
Diagram of a sagittal section through the brain to show the arrangement of association fibers between anterior and posterior regions.
a, b, c: pyramidal cells; *d:* axon terminal arborization; *e:* ascending arborizations of association fiber collaterals; *f:* longitudinal section through the corpus callosum.

giant pyramidal cells. These observations may depend on the fact that it is relatively easy to trace the axon of cells that lie near the white matter.

In most cases these axons simply bend at the level of the white matter to continue as association fibers, although T-shaped divisions with branches of equal or unequal size may also be found (figure 14, *c*). In the latter case, the medial branch may be incorporated into the region of callosal fibers. In any event it appears quite likely, based on the different course and termination of the two branches, that an association fiber can allow a single cell in one part of the cortex or another to contact a large number of other cells in other regions of the same hemisphere, perhaps even in different lobes.

The number of association fibers appears to increase in proportion to the volume of gray matter. Thus association fibers in humans and large mammals, whose gray matter forms gyri, make up the largest component of the white matter due to their numbers. The sheer number and extraordinary length of these fibers, combined with the fact that they intermingle with projection and callosal fibers, renders the anatomical pursuit of any one fiber utterly impossible. It is thus essential to observe small brains (of the rat, bat, mouse, and so on), not only because distances are relatively short, but also because here the association, commissural, and projection fiber systems can be found in certain well-defined regions.

Association Fiber Collaterals   Application of the Golgi method to small and newborn mammals led us to the important discovery that many association fibers give rise to very thin collaterals that ascend and ramify in the overlying cortical gray matter (figure 14, *e*). These fibers are particularly well displayed in certain regions such as the medial face of the hemisphere, where several collaterals can be seen to reach the molecular zone itself and end freely as extended arborizations, an arrangement that is also clear in the reptilian cerebral cortex. In addition to these radial collaterals that end in the gray matter, it is possible to observe collaterals that appear to end in the white matter or in the deepest part of the gray matter. Their orientation is less regular than the radial collaterals, and they appear to establish connections with the many descending dendrites that end within the depths of the white matter. These white matter collaterals appear to be similar to the peripheral collaterals in amphibians and reptiles that ramify among the branches of a perimedullary dendritic plexus.

Association fibers end in the same way as fibers in the white matter of the spinal cord. In other words, they give rise to freely ending arborizations that are so extensive that they invade virtually all parts of the gray matter, including the molecular zone (figure 14, *a*).

Callosal Fibers (figure 15, A)   These fibers lie beneath the association fibers, and in small mammals aggregate in a well-defined layer that forms the roof of the lateral ventricles. In good silver chromate preparations of the corpus callosum, these fibers are immediately obvious because of their extreme

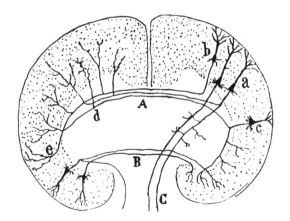

Figure 15
Diagram of transverse section through the brain to show the probable arrangement of commissural and projection fiber.
A: corpus callosum; B: anterior commissure; C: the pyramidal tract, which consists of projection fibers.

delicacy; they appear to be simple axon collaterals. In Weigert-Pal preparations they also display a well defined myelin sheath. Callosal fibers arise in all parts of the cerebral cortex on one side, except in the sphenoidal region, where the commissural fibers form a separate bundle that courses through the anterior commissure (figure 15, B). In addition, some types of callosal fibers appear to bifurcate, with the commissural fiber proceeding along its original horizontal course and the other fiber entering the gray matter (figure 15, *d*).

In transverse sections through the newborn rat brain, where silver chromate preferentially stains callosal fibers, it is possible to observe very fine collaterals that tend to arise and behave very much like those from association fibers. In general, each callosal fiber supplies two or, at most, three such fibers, which arise at nearly right angles, ascend, and become lost in the gray matter, where they end freely.

What is the origin of callosal fibers? Do they represent the direct continuation of axons or are they the collaterals of fibers in the white matter? Or, using the ventral commissure of the spinal cord as an example, is it possible that the corpus callosum harbors direct axons as well as collaterals from axons in the white matter?

The latter view is consistent with my own observations. In fact, many parts of the white matter contain association and projection axons that issue a fine collateral that enters the corpus callosum. Occasionally, more than a collateral is involved; here the fiber destined for the corpus callosum appears to arise at a bifurcation point.

On the other hand, it is not uncommon to observe fibers arising in different layers of the gray matter, particularly at the level of the small pyramidal cells, which descend and then curve sharply to enter the corpus callosum directly. These fibers, which resemble axons, may constitute the direct continuations of the functional processes of small cortical cells. Let me hasten to add, however, that I have not yet been able to confirm this interpretation directly.

How do these callosal fibers end? The answer is still obscure, despite extensive study. I have occasionally observed callosal fibers that climb through the gray matter and ramify, but unfortunately have never been able to follow the terminal branches (figure 15, *e*). It will therefore be necessary to initiate further work on this problem.

In summary, it is my opinion that callosal fibers do not merely unite symmetrical regions in the two hemispheres, as previously thought. Instead, they form a complex transverse association system in which, for example, a fiber that arises from one point in the hemisphere contacts cells in the symmetrical region of the opposite hemisphere, as well as (by way of collaterals) many other elements in different regions and layers of the cortex.

Fibers That Ramify in the Gray Matter (figure 16, E)   As pointed out above, association fibers from distant regions of the same hemisphere enter the gray matter and ramify within it. In addition, there are a number of much thicker fibers that arise in the spinal cord, cerebellum, and other regions and typically course obliquely or horizontally through the gray matter; there they form an immense plexus throughout the thickness of the gray matter, including the molecular zone. The terminal branches form varicose arborizations that appear to surround the small pyramidal cells preferentially. Do these fibers perhaps represent the cerebral endings of sensory nerves, or, at the very least, the axon terminals of cells receiving inputs from the terminal branches of sensory nerves? This seems likely, but has not yet been confirmed. In any event, these fibers are quite readily stained in reptiles, where their principal arborizations are condensed in the molecular zone.

Connections of Cells in the First Layer of the Cerebral Cortex
We saw earlier that all pyramidal cells give rise to a dendritic tuft or bouquet in the molecular zone, which also contains the terminals of innumerable nerve fibers. This dendritic-axonal plexus, which must be quite important since it is found in the

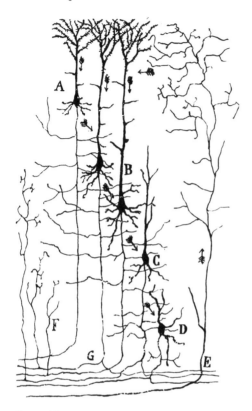

Figure 16
The probable direction of current flow and the pattern of axodendritic connections between cells in the cerebral cortex.
A: small pyramidal cell; B: large pyramidal cell; C and D: polymorph cells; E: terminal fiber arising in another center; F: white matter collaterals; G: an axon that bifurcates in the white matter.

cerebral cortex of all vertebrates, allows pyramidal cells to receive inputs from a great many cells. Let me state at the outset that I believe that these connections are established through the contact of terminal arborizations and axon collaterals from one hemisphere with cell bodies and dendrites in the other. Thus, current flow is *cellulifugal* in the axon, and *cellulipetal* in the cell body and dendrites (Cajal, van Gehuchten), that is, the dendrites and cell body always receive currents, whereas the collaterals and terminal branches of axons transmit current.

These premises have allowed me to interpret the connections of the first layer of the cerebral cortex, the molecular zone. In this zone, the terminal tufts of pyramidal cells are in a position to receive currents from: (1) the axonal ramifications of cells endogenous to the molecular zone; (2) the superficial arborization of the ascending axon of vertical fusiform cells in the cortex; (3) the ascending collaterals and terminal arborizations of the axon from pyramidal association cells in regions more or less removed from the terminal field; (4) the widespread arborizations throughout the cortical gray matter of certain large fibers in the white matter that may arise in the cerebellum, spinal cord, and other regions; and (5) the terminal branches of callosal fibers that may arise in the opposite hemisphere.

Connections at the Level of the Pyramidal and Polymorph Cell Zones
These connections are extremely complex and are established between the cell body, shaft, and dendrites of cells in one hemisphere, and five types of nerve fiber from the other hemisphere. These fiber types include collaterals from the white matter, collaterals from the corpus callosum, terminals of interlobar or extracentral association fibers, axonal arborizations of Golgi (sensory) cells, and finally, vast numbers of collaterals arising from the axons of cells in the three deeper layers as they pass through the gray matter. The plexus formed around these cells by so many different fiber types is so complex that

it would be foolhardy to pretend that all of the connections of
a pyramidal cell can be specified.

Let me simply point out that the fiber plexus probably allows
pyramidal cells to be influenced by: (1) short-axoned cells
(Golgi cells) in the pyramidal layer; (2) association cells in
different lobes of the hemisphere; (3) cells in the opposite
hemisphere (by way of callosal fibers or fibers in the ventral
commissure); (4) cells in the sensory sphere; and (5) giant cells
in more superficial layers of the same cortical region (figure
16).

The connections established by giant cells are surely one of
the most important, and appear to involve the collaterals of
more superficial pyramidal cells that end on the soma, dendritic shaft, and basal dendrites of deeper pyramidal cells.
Each collateral is quite long, branches out, and runs more or
less horizontally. Because of this arrangement it may contact
transversely the dendritic shafts and somata of hundreds of
cells. Thus, the collaterals of a single small pyramidal cell can
influence several series of medium to small pyramidal cells
below it. Similarly, each large pyramidal cell can receive currents from a great many superficial pyramidal cells because of
the huge surface area of its apical and basal dendrites (figure
16, A, B, C, D).

According to the above-mentioned hypothesis of dynamic
polarization for the cellular processes, currents in the cortical
gray matter should flow from the small pyramidal cells to the
large pyramidal cells, and then from the large pyramidal cells
to the polymorph cells, as shown by the arrows in figure 16.

If we knew the mode of termination of sensory nerve fibers
from the spinal cord or other centers closer to the cortex, it
would be possible to establish with greater precision where
currents responsible for voluntary movement begin in the projection cells. Despite my ignorance on this interesting topic,
there is no lack of ideas about how to construct hypotheses.
For example, sensory nerve fibers or fibers in sensory pathways always end freely as arborizations in the molecular layer
of the cortex (or in an equivalent layer in other nerve centers

like the cortical layer of the avian optic lobe), where they contact the peripheral dendritic tufts of elongated cells. This arrangement is particularly obvious in the mammalian olfactory lobe; many fibers from the olfactory bulb send collateral and terminal branches to a superficial zone where they contact the dendritic bouquets of pyramidal cells, just as in the molecular layer of the cerebral cortex. In the reptilian cerebral cortex as well, olfactory fibers along with all of the deep axons (which probably include sensory fibers from the spinal cord) tend to ramify in the superficial or molecular layer.

These and other considerations lead me to believe that the initiation of voluntary movements begins at the tuft or dendritic bouquet of pyramidal cells, and is thus generated in the molecular zone. This would explain why physiologists may induce movements in particular groups of muscles after subjecting the cerebral cortex to mechanical, chemical, or electrical stimulation. The diffuse excitation of the molecular zone could act directly on the tuft of pyramidal cells or, as seems less likely, indirectly on the nerve fibers in this zone that are in intimate contact with these tufts. In this way, the stimulus would act at the same point as the will of the experimental animal.

Morphological Classification of Cerebral Cells
Anatomists have always been preoccupied with the question of how to deduce the function of the various morphological features of neurons. Thus, Golgi presumed that nerve centers contain two cell types that differ in their morphology and physiology: one class gives rise to axons that ramify immediately, losing their individuality in the process, while the other gives rise to axons that maintain their individuality as far as the white matter, although they give rise to collaterals in the gray matter. He regarded the first type of cell as sensory because the axonal branches intermingle with the plexus formed by centripetal fibers, whereas the second type were considered motor cells because the axons enter the motor roots.

However, this classification has not found support on morphological or physiological grounds, as Koelliker, His, Waldeyer, van Gehuchten, and others have pointed out.

Morphologically, the first type (sensory cell) only differs from the second (motor cell) with regard to the length of its axon. The axon of the former is short and remains entirely within the gray matter, where it arborizes into freely ending terminals near its origin. In contrast, the functional process of the second type is long, and courses through the white matter before arborizing in other nerve centers or in organs outside the central nervous system. In view of this, I have referred to Golgi's two cell types as short-axoned and long-axoned cells, a nomenclature that has been adopted by many authors because it implies nothing about underlying cellular physiology.

Golgi's classification is not supported by physiological considerations, either. Obvious sensory organs like the retina, olfactory bulb, olfactory mucosa, and so on, contain long-axoned cells (Golgi motor cells), whereas organs that are clearly influenced by the motor sphere, such as the cerebellum and the psychomotor region of the cerebral cortex, contain many short-axoned cells.

There are actually three morphologically distinct cell types in the cerebral cortex: (1) short-axoned cells (Golgi sensory cells, polygonal cells, and some fusiform cells in the first layer); (2) long-axoned cells (pyramidal cells, polymorph cells, and so on); and (3) special cells with axon-like processes (bipolar and triangular cells in the first layer). The third type is also found in amphibians and reptiles. The cells in this category are unusual in that all of their processes are thick as they leave the cell body, and then gradually assume the appearance of nerve fibers as they ramify. If we can demonstrate in mammals (which we have not yet been able to do) that the dendrite-like processes of these fusiform and triangular cells end as thin axon-like fibers, then the brain is similar to the retina and olfactory bulb, where the two principal cell types are joined by a third in which axons and dendrites cannot be distinguished.

In summary, it is not possible at this time to attach a particular functional modality (such as sensory, motor, commissural, or associative) to particular morphological classes of nerve cells. Furthermore, the same restriction applies, with some qualifications, to the various layers of the cerebral cortex. Thus, commissural, association, and projection cells are not confined to one layer or another, but instead are intermingled in all of the layers. This arrangement may help to explain why intellectual impairments are rarely limited to one sphere of activity, and why cerebral functions are often retained after a serious lesion to one or another cortical region.

The Cerebral Cortex of Lower Vertebrates

Reptiles

Edinger has pointed out that among the lower vertebrates (birds, reptiles, amphibians, fish), only reptiles display a cortex similar to that of mammals. The following layers may be observed in the anterior vesicle of *Lacerta agilis* (figure 17), a representative reptile.

1. The molecular layer   As in mammals, this layer contains three elements: (*a*) the terminal bouquets of pyramidal cells; (*b*) the horizontal processes of certain fusiform or globular cells, comparable to special cells in the mammalian molecular layer; and (*c*) the terminal arborizations of a great many nerve fibers, some of which are collaterals or axon terminals from the white matter and others that are the ascending collaterals of axons from cells in the gray matter.

2. The pyramidal cell layer   This layer contains several compact series of cells that are either fusiform, triangular, or pyramidal in shape. The dendrites of these cells ramify in the molecular zone, while the axons enter the white matter.

3. Plexiform layer   This layer contains a few large pyramidal cells that are quite similar to those in the second layer. However, the plexiform layer is dominated by a vast number of nerve fibers that form a dense plexus.

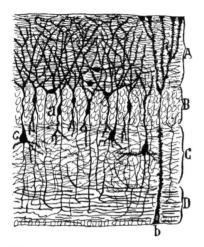

Figure 17
Section of the *Lacerta agilis* cerebral cortex.
A: molecular or superficial plexiform layer; B: pyramidal cell layer;
C: molecular or deep (inner) plexiform layer; *a:* pyramidal cell; *b:* epithelial
cell; *c:* pyramidal cell of the inner plexiform layer.

4. The layer of white matter   Callosal, projection, and perhaps
even association fibers can be observed in this layer. As P.
Ramon first noted, the neuroglia are represented by radiating
epithelial cells that lie next to the ventricle and end as a tuft
of spiny filaments at the very surface of the brain.

Amphibia
Work in the amphibian cerebral cortex by Oyarsum, Edinger,
and myself has demonstrated that while the cellular morphology is comparable to that seen in mammals, the number of
layers and the course of the nerve fibers are not (figure 18).
   In the frog, for example, there are only two well-defined
neural layers. As in reptiles and mammals, the molecular or
superficial zone contains the following structural elements: a
collection of spiny tufts from pyramidal cells; horizontal cell
processes that do not form distinct axons and/or dendrites;

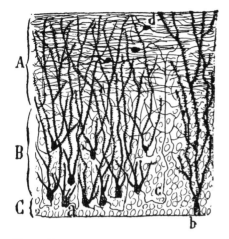

Figure 18
A section through the cerebral cortex of a frog.
A: molecular layer; B: pyramidal cell layer; C: epithelial layer; *a:* the soma of
a pyramidal cell that gives rise to an ascending axon *(c); d:* a cell in the
molecular layer; *b:* an epithelial cell with ramifications that extend just deep
to the pia mater.

and finally, the terminal arborizations of a great many ascending nerve fibers. The pyramidal cell zone occupies the deep half of the cortex. The vast majority of primary axons derived from cells in this zone are ascending, and ramify within the molecular zone.

Oyarsum also observed pyramidal cells that give rise to a caudally directed axon, which may well constitute a projection fiber. However, this cell type is not found in all parts of the anterior vesicle, being absent in dorsal regions of the hemispheres.

In addition to pyramidal cells with an ascending axon, Calleja recently observed Golgi sensory cells whose short arborizations form a plexus between pyramidal cell bodies and part of the adjacent molecular layer.

Do the pyramidal cells in the frog correspond to a particular cell type in the mammalian cortex? In my opinion they may be considered association cells with a short axon that ascends to nearby parts of the molecular layer, where its thin arborizations contact many pyramidal cells, rather than cells with a long axon that courses horizontally to neighboring regions of the ventricular cavity. Commissural cells appear to be absent in the frog cerebral cortex, and projection cells are only found in ventral parts of the anterior vesicle.

The neuroglia has been described in detail by Oyarsum. As in reptiles, it consists of epithelial cells with a large bouquet of distal ramifications that end below the pia mater by way of conical expansions (figure 18, *b*).

Birds
Recent work by Cl. Sala indicates that the cerebral cortex of birds (the supraventricular region) is no more advanced than that of reptiles. In fact, the avian cortex appears to be more like that of amphibians than that of reptiles; there is no layer of white matter, cells with an ascending axon predominate, and commissural cells are absent. It consists of three layers: (1) a molecular layer; (2) a layer of small and large pyramidal cells, and (3) a layer of stellate cells (figure 19).

The structure of the molecular layer is the same as in reptiles and amphibians. It is formed by a combination of ascending nerve fibers, the dendrites of pyramidal cells, and the pseudo-axons of certain globular or fusiform special cells.

The pyramidal cell layer consists of several series of more or less elongated cells giving rise to ascending and descending dendrites. The ascending processes extend into the molecular layer, whereas the descending dendrites ramify within the third. The axon of these cells may ramify immediately to end freely between the somata of nearby pyramidal cells, and it may also climb toward the molecular zone, where it gives rise to a luxuriant arborization. A few of these cells give rise to an axon that courses vertically through the interhemispheric part of the cortex to end, along with many other fibers, in a deep, dorsoventrally oriented bundle that may form a projection system; this is the tract of the wall of the longitudinal

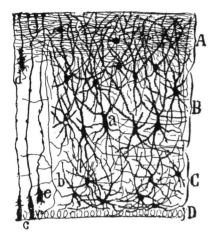

Figure 19
Section through the cerebral cortex of a newborn chick at the level of the supraventricular region, based on preparations by Cl. Sala
A: molecular layer; B: pyramidal cell layer; C: stellate cell layer (corresponding to the mammalian polymorph cells); D: epithelium; *a:* pyramidal cell; *b:* stellate cell with an ascending axon; *c:* epithelial cells; *d, e:* displaced epithelial cells that have migrated and are in the process of developing into spider cells.

fissure or what the Germans describe as *Bündeln der sagittalen Scheidewand*.

The stellate cell layer lies adjacent to the epithelium. Stellate cell dendrites course in all directions without extending into the molecular zone. The axon of many of these cells is like that of Golgi sensory cells because it ramifies between the somata of pyramidal cells and neighboring stellate cells, although occasional branches extend as far as the molecular zone.

Structure-Function Relationships
The following psychophysiological considerations emerge from the above discussion of the arrangement of psychic cells.

1. Given our current state of knowledge, neither the external morphology of psychic cells nor the connections between

them are sufficient to explain the supreme role played by cortical activity. Morphological differences between these cells and the typical nerve cell are hardly noticeable, and are readily explained by the vast richness of the connections established by every psychic cell. In fact all nerve cells, regardless of their function, appear to be constructed from the same model, with the same texture and chemical composition. Motor cells in the ventral horn of the spinal cord, ganglion cells in the retina, cells in the sympathetic chain of vertebrates, and so on, all display the same axon, the same dendrites, and the same mode of establishing contacts and transmitting currents. In short, neurons in general exhibit all of the features character-istic of psychic cells, although we attribute to the latter the highest activities of life including the association of ideas, memory, and intelligence. From the standpoint of the com-plexity of its connections and the variety of its morphologically distinct cell types, the cerebral cortex does not even rival the cerebellum and retina; however the activities of these organs, no matter how important, must be considered crude when compared to the specific functions of the cerebral cortex. To avoid becoming discouraged by the battle to understand this immensely complex problem, and to accommodate the strong inclination to explain thought in mechanical terms, science would do well to consider the possibility that the "something" that distinguishes cerebral cells from cells in the brain stem, spinal cord, and ganglia is not based on external form but rather on architectural details and chemical composition, and that activity in the protoplasm of psychic cells is not even remotely equivalent to that in lower nerve cells.

2. Another conclusion that can be drawn from considera-tions of structure-function relationships, and one that many anatomists have arrived at and that has been defended bril-liantly by Letamendi, is that there is no one receptive center for all types of sensory fibers and no one source for all of the motor fibers. Instead, the cerebral cortex as a whole may be regarded as a series of centers, each receiving a particular type of sensory fiber and influencing a particular type of motor

fiber. These centers are interconnected by way of association and commissural fiber systems, which allow the formation of a variety of mental (as well as conscious and unconscious sensory-motor) associations. These special cortical zones do not have a particular texture that would serve to explain this specific function. As Golgi noted, functional specificity in the cortex derives from a much earlier stage, namely, from the special peripheral connections (with sensory organs, muscles, and so on) of the fibers that are related to one of these cortical centers.

3. With few exceptions, it seems clear that psychic functions are correlated with the presence of pyramidal (psychic) cells throughout the animal kingdom. As Edinger recently pointed out, fish show no sign of intellectual capacity, and true pyramidal cells are absent in their ventral cerebral vesicles.

The pyramidal or psychic cell displays a number of features that are invariably present in amphibians, reptiles, birds, and mammals. The most obvious features include the presence of a shaft and dendritic bouquet (or tuft) that course vertically toward the surface of the brain, and the existence of collateral spines, all of which are connected to a dense plexus of nerve fiber terminals at the level of the molecular layer (see figure 12).

4. Pyramidal cells are elongated and give rise to a variety of different processes so that they may be influenced by a large number of different types of cellular elements. Just as the cerebellar Purkinje cell is highly differentiated, with each of its parts (the cell body, primary shaft, and dendrites) in contact with nerve fibers of different origin, so the pyramidal cells also become highly elongated; thus nerve fibers that may arise in different centers may influence the cell body, the basilar processes, the shaft, and the terminal tuft. Thus, the degree to which the dendritic arborization is differentiated allows us to estimate the number of distinct types of input to a particular cell.

5. Because the psychic cell becomes progressively larger and more complex in ascending the animal scale, it is only natural

to assume that at least part of its increased functional role is a result of increased morphological complexity. It is possible that this increase is not related to the essence of psychic behaviors, but is instead related to their extent and content.

It therefore seems likely that the activity of psychic cells is dispersed more widely and usefully because of the large number of dendrites, somatic processes, and collaterals they give rise to, and because their axon gives rise to more collaterals, which are longer and ramify more frequently. Although the size of a nerve cell may occasionally be correlated with its developmental stage, this is often not the case. In general, the volume of a nerve cell appears to be proportional to the size of the animal. For example, pyramidal cells in the chicken and lizard are larger than in the sparrow and wall lizard, respectively. In spite of this size difference, however, they are no more or no less differentiated, and are thus incapable of elaborating higher intellectual activity. It should also be pointed out that the size of the cell body is proportional to the extent and richness of branching in the terminal arborizations of its axon. In other words, the larger the cell, the more cells (whether neural, glandular, muscle, or other) it can contact. Neither the length of the axon nor the richness of its dendritic arbors appears to influence consistently the size of the cell body.

6. The psychic cell begins ontogenetic development as a simple neuroblast, that is, as a piriform cell with only one process, the axon. It then becomes more complex with the formation of a bud for the primary apical process; finally the lateral branches of the shaft, cell body, and axon appear.

7. Based on the fact that the space between psychic cells contains axonal and dendritic arborizations, it is possible to infer the extent of psychic cell differentiation by measuring the distance between them. Thus, psychic cells in amphibians and reptiles almost come in contact with one another in many areas, whereas in humans they are widely separated.

The general principle that I have just elaborated, namely that the functional importance of a cell is directly related to the

number of its axon collaterals, may help explain two observations that are difficult to interpret in light of the generally
accepted hypothesis that intelligence is related directly to the
actual number of cortical cells, which are a simple instrument
of the soul, or an exclusive substrate for psychic activity. One
is the remarkable intellectual growth seen in people devoted
to continuous, deep mental exercise, and the other is the
expression of outstanding talent, even true genius, in brains
that are average or below average in volume and weight.

In the first instance, we may postulate that cerebral gym-
nastics push the development of axon collaterals and dendrites
slightly further than usual, thus establishing new, more extensive intercortical connections. This conclusion is based on the
fact that new cells cannot be produced; nerve cells do not
multiply like muscle cells. During this process, there may be
a concomitant decrease in the size of neuronal cell bodies or
the glial framework around them to maintain a constant volume of cerebral tissue.   In the second instance, there is no
reason to doubt that certain brains compensate for a small
number of cells by developing a larger number of collaterals,
either because previous adaptations have been inherited or for
other reasons.

Naturally, these explanations are based on a logical hypothesis about the role played by cells and their processes. It is
necessary to assume that each active psychic cell captures a
simple image (in some as yet unknown oscillatory or chemical
form) of each sensory impression, whether from the outside
world or from the tissues of our own organs (for example, the
muscle sense).

Thus, whatever the nature of higher activity may be that
associates, judges, compares, and so on, only the axon and
dendrites of nerve cells can form the pathways underlying
these processes.

If, as Bain claims, to *understand* is to perceive the similarities
and differences between our ideas, then the richness and
breadth of judgment would be even greater, since there would
be a larger storehouse of acquired images for the cellular sub-

strate of the brain to establish a more highly developed system of relationships.

These considerations apply only to certain properties of psychic acts, not to their essential nature, which no hypothesis has yet explained adequately. Neither materialism nor spiritualism can explain how an impulse arriving in the first layer of the cerebral cortex is converted into something as different as an act of conscience.

Both hypotheses provide relatively satisfactory explanations for the union and continuity between the sensory and motor spheres. According to the spiritualist doctrine, the soul acts as a receptor organ in one part of the brain and as an impulse generating organ in another part, somewhat like the telegraph operator who is stationed at a central location to receive and transmit orders over multiple lines simultaneously. The system of material interrelationships established between motor and sensory pathways is responsible only for brain automatisms; the soul itself is the unifying arch for conscious phenomena.

According to the materialist hypothesis, the same events take place except that the conscious chain established between centripetal and centrifugal stimuli is mediated by a very special action, the transformation of sensory activity into motor activity, rather than by the intervention of an immaterial, destructive movement generator. Thus there would be no interruption of current flow between the two ends of the conscious arch, but rather a simple reflection of currents associated with the various modalities. The nature, extent, and complexity of the motor response elicited by the reception of a sensory stimulus, as well as the registration of a conceptual representation or idea, would thus be an inevitable consequence of the anatomical organization of the cortical receptive areas. It would appear that each of these areas contains a group of related cells for the reception of impressions, as well as a subordinate group of projection or excitomotor cells.

Chapter 4
Ammon's Horn

A number of classical treatises on Ammon's horn have been written by Kupffer, Meinert, Krause, Duval, Giaccomini, and others, in addition to the work done on this region by Golgi, L. Sala, and Schaeffer, who favored the silver chromate method. In order to complete the cycle of my own work on the structure of the nervous system, I have also carried out a series of studies on Ammon's horn in the rabbit and guinea pig using the Golgi-Cox method and the double impregnation method, which is simply my own modification of the rapid Golgi method. The following is a brief summary of these results.

It is well known that Ammon's horn consists of two adjacent cortical gyri that are relatively simple in structure and are interrelated so that the molecular layer of one (the dentate gyrus, or embossed body) is continuous with that of the other (Ammon's horn).

Given the structural similarities between the cerebral cortex and these gyri, it should not be surprising that the same layers are found in both. These layers include the (1) white matter, (2) polymorph cell layer, (3) pyramidal cell layer, and (4) molecular or plexiform layer.

Ammon's Horn Proper

1. White Matter (alveus)
The white matter is formed by the axons of pyramidal cells and different types of polymorph cells (Sala, Schaeffer). In general, these fibers give rise to only a few collaterals during

their horizontal course, except in that part of the alveus bordering the hilus of the dentate gyrus, where a very large number of collaterals may be observed.

The ramified processes of ependymal cells are found between the fiber bundles of the alveus in the newborn rabbit. Some of these processes are so long that they extend into the superficial part of the molecular zone, where their thin, varicose branches invade a wide area.

2. Polymorph Cell Layer

The cells in this layer were noted by Sala and described perfectly by Schaeffer, who also clarified the course and other features of their axon (figure 20, *b, d,* and *e*).

a. The deepest part of this zone contains fusiform cells that are oriented parallel to the fibers in the *alveus.* The dendrites of these cells branch among the myelinated fibers of the alveus, and it appears to me that the axon of at least some of these cells behaves like that of the so-called Golgi sensory cell; that is, the parent axon ascends toward the surface and quickly disappears following extensive ramification.

b. The superficial or outer part of the polymorph cell layer is much thicker and displays features characteristic of a plexiform zone. It is within this region that the basal dendrites of pyramidal cells come into contact with axon collaterals from the very same cells. According to Schaeffer, this part of the polymorph layer also contains three other special cell types, with either an ascending, a descending, or a horizontal axon.

The cells with an ascending axon were discovered and drawn by Schaeffer, who distinguished two subtypes on the basis of the way in which their axon behaves.

The first type consists primarily of fusiform or triangular cells in superficial parts of the polymorph layer. They display both ascending and descending dendrites, and their axon ascends, giving rise to several branches in the most superficial part of the stratum radiatum. However, the parent axons then descend, like the collaterals they issue at right angles as they ascend through the stratum radiatum, all the way to the py-

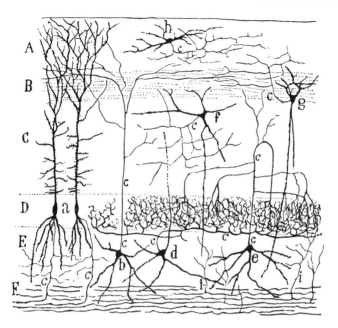

Figure 20
Section through Ammon's horn of an eight-day-old rabbit.
A: stratum moleculare; B: stratum lacunosum; C: stratum radiatum;
D: pyramidal cell layer; E: polymorph cell layer; F: white matter or *alveus;*
a: pyramidal cell; *b:* cell with an ascending axon; *d:* cell with a horizontal axon
that ramifies between pyramidal cell perikarya; *e:* cell with an arching axon
that ends in the interpyramidal plexus; *f:* short-axoned cell in the stratum
radiatum; *g:* cell in the stratum lacunosum; *h:* cell in the stratum moleculare.
Axonal processes are indicated by a *c.*

ramidal cell layer, where they dissolve into an extraordinarily rich pericellular plexus that consists of highly varicose terminal branches. Thus, the axon of this cell type consistently follows an arching course to the pyramidal layer that is concave relative to the deep white matter. The plexus that these axons form in the pyramidal layer also receives contributions from other sources (cells with a horizontal axon), and represents one of the most important structural features of Ammon's horn, although I seem to have been the first to have observed it. Because of this arrangement, each cell with an ascending axon may contact a considerable number of pyramidal cells, and even a few cells in the superficialmost part of the molecular zone (figure 20, *e*).

The second type was described quite well by Schaeffer; the ascending axon ramifies in the molecular and lacunar (stratum lacunosum) layers, but does not issue descending branches (figure 20, *b*).

The cells with a descending axon are fusiform or triangular in shape and represent displaced pyramidal cells; the axon of these cells enters the *alveus*.

The cells with a horizontal axon (figure 20, *d*) are stellate and quite large. They are found throughout the superficial part of the polymorph layer, although they are more abundant in the region nearest the pyramidal cell zone. These elements fall into the category of Golgi sensory cells, and were probably observed by L. Sala and Schaeffer. It is important to point out that the most interesting feature of these cells is the course and branching pattern of their axon, which travels in a horizontal or slightly ascending direction and divides into several large, varicose branches that course in different directions, always skirting the pyramidal layer. These large varicose branches are occasionally very long and give rise along their course to ascending collaterals that enter the pyramidal layer, where they form a very dense plexus of short, varicose, rather granular twigs around the pyramidal cells. As described above, the descending branches of the cells with an ascending axon (the first type) also contribute to this plexus.

3. The Pyramidal Cell Layer

The pyramidal cells of Ammon's horn have long been recognized because of their large volume and pyramidal shape. They were examined very carefully by Golgi, who succeeded in staining them with his black impregnation method; Sala and Schaeffer added some further details to his description (figure 20, *a*).

In the rabbit and guinea pig, these cells display an oval or fusiform rather than a pyramidal shape, and are arranged in three or more superimposed rows. As Schaeffer pointed out, the deepest, or inner row contains the largest pyramidal cells.

The roots or descending dendrites arise from the deep pole of the cell body, whereas the superficial pole gives rise to a radial shaft that gives rise to several collaterals as it passes through the stratum radiatum, and then dissolves into a bouquet of varicose, spiny branches at the level of the stratum lacunosum. The collateral spines, which were described by Schaeffer, are a unique feature that places these bouquets in the same category as those found on pyramidal cells in the cerebral cortex. The dendritic branches of the bouquet reach the most superficial part of the molecular layer, where they show no particular preference for blood vessels or neuroglial cells, as held by Golgi and Sala (figure 20, A).

The axons descend to the alveus, where they often simply bend and then continue as myelinated fibers. However, some axons bifurcate in a Y-shape upon entering the white matter, and in the process give rise to a thick and a thin fiber, both of which continue as nerve fibers in the alveus. It is possible that the thinner fiber, which usually courses in a direction opposite to that of the thicker fiber, enters the Ammonic commissure along with many other analogous fibers. This commissure consists of a bundle of thin fibers below the corpus callosum that interconnects the dorsal end of Ammon's horn on one side of the brain with the corresponding region on the opposite side. As it descends, the pyramidal cell axon gives rise to two or more collaterals that ramify and disappear within the thickness of the polymorph layer. These collaterals were described previously by Golgi and Sala.

The most salient general features of ammonic pyramidal cells have just been described. However, it is also important to note that pyramidal cells in the *regio inferior* of Ammon's horn (which lies adjacent to and below the *fimbria*) are not identical to those in the *regio superior*. The major differences are as follows:

1. It is well known that pyramidal cells in the *regio inferior* are larger than those in the *regio superior,* and that they have a short, thick vertical shaft with a dendritic bouquet that might be regarded as arising prematurely.

2. The axons of pyramidal cells in the *regio inferior* enter the fimbria and then the fornix, whereas at least some of the functional processes of cells in the *regio superior* course to the white matter of the subiculum (the bed of Ammon's horn) and then give rise to freely ending arborizations in the gray matter of this cortical region. That is, it would appear that cells in the *regio inferior* give rise to a system of projection fibers, while cells in the *regio superior* give rise to a system of association fibers.

3. Schaeffer discovered that the thick axon of inferior or giant pyramidal cells gives rise to one or occasionally two thick collaterals that ascend to the stratum lacunosum and then course horizontally through the entire length of the *regio superior,* where they ramify to contact the apical bouquet of small pyramidal cells (fig. 22, H). Ascending collaterals do not arise directly from the axon of superior cells, at least along their descending course.

4. The soma and initial part of the vertical shaft of small pyramidal cells in the *regio superior* are smooth, and it is only in the stratum radiatum that the shaft begins to display a few thin collateral spines. In contrast the shaft, and occasionally even adjacent parts of the soma, of *regio inferior* pyramidal cells appears to be invested with thick, ramified excrescences. Mossy fibers (which are the axons of granule cells in the fascia

dentata) and their collateral rosettes become lodged in notches in these excrescences.

5. As we shall see later, from the dynamic point of view the large pyramidal cells are associated with granule cells, while the small (superior) pyramidal cells are not, as shown schematically in figure 22.

4. Molecular or Plexiform Layer

Because it is particularly thick and harbors a variety of components, it is convenient to divide this layer into three subzones: deep (stratum radiatum), middle (stratum lacunosum), and superficial (stratum moleculare).

a. Deep subzone (stratum radiatum or radiated layer) (figure 20, C). This zone occupies more than half the thickness of the plexiform layer and contains the dendritic shafts of pyramidal and other cell types in deeper layers, as well as an extremely rich plexus of nerve fibers. However, it also contains a number of special cell types, the most common of which include the following.

1. Displaced pyramidal cells, which are elongated and display a variety of shapes. Nevertheless, the dendrites and axon of these cells behave just as those of the large pyramidal cells.

2. Large triangular or stellate cells with very long, varicose processes that frequently display a horizontal or oblique orientation. The axon of these cells runs for a short distance parallel or obliquely to the molecular layer and gives rise to a widely distributed arborization of thin, granular fibers that are essentially straight and concentrated in distinct planes of the molecular layer.

3. Triangular or fusiform cells with a descending axon that gives rise to freely ending arborizations around pyramidal cell somata, and invades the polymorph cell zone as well.

4. The deep zone contains fusiform or stellate cells with an axon that ascends to the stratum lacunosum and stratum moleculare and cannot be followed any farther.

All of these cell types give rise to ascending dendrites in the stratum lacunosum and stratum moleculare, as well as descending dendrites in the polymorph cell layer (figure 20, *f*).

b. Middle subzone (stratum lacunosum or lacunar layer). This subzone contains nerve cells as well as bundles of myelinated fibers (figure 20, B).

Most of the cells are triangular in shape and form one or two irregular rows in the deepest part of this subzone. They give rise to ascending as well as descending dendrites, although the former are more common. The axon (figure 20, *g*) courses more or less horizontally through the stratum lacunosum and gives rise to branches that end in this subzone, or in the overlying molecular subzone.

The horizontal bundles consist of fibers that stretch from the inferior region of Ammon's horn to the vicinity of the subiculum. As Schaeffer noted, the majority of such fibers are ascending collaterals derived from the axons of large pyramidal cells in the inferior region of Ammon's horn. The remaining fibers are either the terminal or collateral branches of axons in the white matter, the terminal arborizations of cells with an ascending axon, or are derived from yet other sources.

c. Superficial subzone (stratum moleculare or molecular subzone). This zone contains the most peripheral segments of the pyramidal cell terminal bouquets, as well as a vast array of nerve fibers. The most important classes of the latter include the terminal branches of ascending axons, the terminal arborizations and collaterals of fibers in the white matter, and the ramifications of endogenous cells or of cells in the stratum lacunosum (figure 20, A).

The endogenous cells (figure 20, *h*) are small and may be fusiform, triangular, or stellate in shape. They give rise to a thin axon that may course in any direction before dissolving into a single expansive arborization consisting of slender, varicose fibers. Earlier authors have noted that these fibers course in all directions throughout the thickness of the stratum moleculare. I have only observed special fusiform cells analogous to those in the first layer of the cerebral cortex on two occasions.

Embossed Body or Fascia Dentata

It is convenient at this point to note that I have previously distinguished three layers in this region: (1) a plexiform or molecular layer, (2) a layer of small pyramidal cells (stratum granulosum), and (3) a layer of polymorph cells (zona reticulata, and so on).

1. Molecular or Plexiform Zone

Like molecular zones elsewhere, it contains two classes of intricately interlaced fibers: the spiny dendrites of cells in deeper layers, and axon terminals. In addition, Sala pointed out that it also contains nerve cells, although until quite recently little was known about their features (figure 21, *a, b*).

My own studies have now shown the following two cell types in this zone.

a. Displaced pyramidal or oval cells share all of the features characteristic of cells in the stratum granulosum except that they are triangular or crescent shaped and are found at various levels of the molecular layer. The axon may either descend directly, or it may follow a long, hook-shaped course in the horizontal plane before descending. In either case it continues on as a mossy fiber in the stratum lucidum or suprapyramidal region of Ammon's horn (figure 21, *d*).

b. Short-axoned cells should be divided into superficial and deep types. The superficial cells (figure 21, *a*) are smaller and may be piriform, oval, or fusiform in shape. They have thin dendrites, which usually descend, and a very thin axon that travels for a short distance before ending in the outer part of the molecular zone as a group of short, even thinner branches. The deep cells (figure 21, *b*) are larger, may be either triangular or stellate in shape, and lie within the deep half of the molecular layer. Their dendrites spread in three directions and not uncommonly pass through the granular zone to end in the

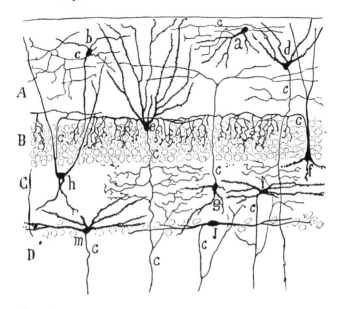

Figure 21
The layers of the fascia dentata in the eight-day-old rabbit.
A: molecular layer; B: granule cell layer; C: polymorph cell layer; D: molecular layer of Ammon's horn; *a, b:* cells of the molecular layer; *d:* displaced granule cell; *e:* granule cell; *f:* pyramidal cell with an ascending axon; *h:* cell with an ascending axon that contributes to the supra- and intergranular neural plexus; *g:* cell with an ascending axon that ramifies in the molecular layer; *i, j, m:* cells with a descending axon that enters the alveus. These axonal processes are indicated by *c.*

polymorph cell layer. The axon is thicker than that of the superficial cells, and may course in a number of different directions. It generates a great many branches that tend to aggregate in the outer or superficial half of the molecular zone, where they extend horizontally for great distances as they ramify. Sala observed and drew one of these two cell types.

2. Pyramidal Cell Layer (Granular Zone, Stratum Granulosum)
In general, my own studies on the cells in this layer fully confirm the descriptions of Golgi, Sala, and Schaeffer. The majority of such cells are oval, triangular, or crescent shaped and all of the dendrites arise from the superficial aspect of the cell body, that is, from the surface facing the molecular zone. The thin axon follows a descending path and continues on as a gnarled fiber after issuing four, six, or eight thin (or occasionally thick), flexuous collaterals from varicosities at the level of the inner half of the plexiform zone. I have been unable to stain the descending axon of Golgi type-two cells that, according to Sala, end by generating a diffuse plexus in the subjacent polymorph layer. In my opinion, every cell in the granular layer gives rise to an axon that can, under favorable circumstances, be followed all the way to the suprapyramidal region (stratum lucidum) of Ammon's horn (figures 21, *e* and 22, D).

Leaving this problem aside, the bundles of axons derived from granule cells are organized just as those drawn and described by Schaeffer. After reaching a certain point in the suprapyramidal region of Ammon's horn, they assume a horizontal orientation; that is, they are arranged along the length of this organ, all the while maintaining the characteristic knotty appearance first noted by L. Sala. In the newborn or very young rabbit and guinea pig, analogous swellings, which increase in size toward the distal end of the axon, do not look like simple varicosities. Instead, they appear as a focal point for the radiation of either varicose fibers that vary in length, or short, thick processes. In a word, the axons of small pyramidal cells are an exact replica of the mossy fibers I described in the cerebellum. A great deal of thought about the course of

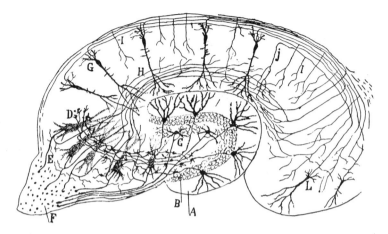

Figure 22
A diagram of Ammon's horn and the fascia dentata to show the relationship between large pyramidal cells of the regio inferior of Ammon's horn and the mossy fibers of granule cells.
A: molecular layer of the fascia dentata; B: granule cell layer; C: molecular layer of the terminal part of Ammon's horn; D: longitudinal bundle of mossy fibers, the axons of granule cells; E: axons of the large pyramidal cells coursing toward the fimbria; F: fimbria; G: small or superior pyramidal cell; H: bundle of large ascending axon collaterals; I: collaterals from the white matter; J: fiber terminals from the subiculum; L: pyramidal cells in the subiculum with an axon that enters Ammon's horn.

granule cell axons, or mossy fibers, leads me to believe that the terminal arborizations contact the soma and shaft of the large pyramidal cells in Ammon's horn (from the inferior part of this organ to a region just above the fimbria).

The following points support this view. (1) A very large proportion of the mossy fibers end freely as either a varicosity or a rosette that contacts the soma or shaft of a large pyramidal cell (figure 22). (2) Mossy fibers never extend beyond the region of the stratum lucidum into the alveus or the stratum lacunosum. Once a mossy fiber enters the layer associated with the large pyramidal cells, it stays there until it ends (figure 22, **D**). (3) Careful examination of the dorsal end of Ammon's horn (along the midline, below the corpus callosum), as well as the ventral end near the border of the sphenoid lobe in the rabbit, guinea pig, and rat, shows exactly the same relationship between mossy fibers and large pyramidal cells. (4) In all parts of Ammon's horn, the edge facing the concavity of the *fascia dentata* can always be shown to contain large pyramidal cells. (5) Mossy fibers and their rosettes become lodged in a unique rough area that is confined to one part of the perikaryon and stem of the large pyramidal cells. (6) Mossy fibers constitute terminal arborizations in the cerebellum. (7) As Sala and Schaeffer first noted, mossy fibers of the fascia dentata lack a myelin sheath, a feature that is typical of axon terminal arborizations.

In addition, the superior part of the granule cell zone contains a few pyramidal cells that are exactly comparable to those found in the cerebral cortex. The deep base of these cells gives rise to several dendrites that branch and end in the subjacent zone, while the superficial process extends through the granule cells as a dendritic shaft that branches in the molecular zone. The axon usually arises from the ascending part of the dendritic shaft, just above the granule cell zone, and courses horizontally while giving off descending ramifications that end among the granule cells. Two axonal plexuses are thus formed: one consists of thick, horizontally oriented fibers in the deep third of the molecular zone that represent a group of axons from pyramidal cells in the granular zone, and the other, which is extremely rich and lies in the outer half of the granular zone, consists of the descending collaterals of this axonal plexus. Thus, each granule cell is literally embedded within a nest or basket of flexuous, varicose axon terminals that completely surrounds it (figure 21, *f*).

Some of these pyramidal cells are also found at deeper levels, in the middle of the polymorph cell zone.

3. Polymorph Cell Layer
The existence of a polymorph layer, similar to that in Ammon's horn, was first noted by Schaeffer, who was able to stain

certain pyramidal or stellate cells with dendrites that enter the molecular zone and an axon that descends into the hilar region. He also observed certain horizontal fusiform cells that had been figured earlier by L. Sala.

I have confirmed the accuracy of these descriptions and have added a number of observations that allow us to understand more clearly the organization of this zone, as well as to compare it with its homolog in Ammon's horn.

It is convenient for descriptive purposes to begin by distinguishing two subzones in the polymorph zone: a superficial or plexiform subzone and a deep subzone with irregular cells. A molecular zone that is related to the large pyramidal cells of Ammon's horn (buried within the hilus of the fascia dentata) lies just below the deep subzone.

A. Plexiform Subzone
In addition to the extremely dense plexus of collaterals mentioned above, this subzone contains a variety of nerve cells that I have divided into three types: (1) cells with an ascending axon; (2) cells with a descending axon; and (3) Golgi sensory cells or short-axoned cells (figure 21.)

1. Cells with an ascending axon are triangular, oval, or stellate in shape. They give rise to one or more dendritic shafts that disappear into the molecular zone, several varicose dendrites that enter the polymorph layer, and an ascending axon that bifurcates at various levels of the molecular zone and then gives rise to a large number of branches that contribute substantially to the axonal plexus in the molecular zone (figure 21, *g*).

Some of these cells behave like the pyramidal cells described earlier; that is, their ascending axon crosses the granule cell layer and then assumes a horizontal course, contributing to the formation of the supragranular and intergranular plexuses mentioned above (figure 21, *h*).

2. The cells with a descending axon usually lie within a deeper plane of the plexiform subzone. They have a tapered

or stellate appearance, and their processes, which are characteristically very long and spiny, generally assume a horizontal course. The large axon of these cells descends as far as the hilar region and then continues into the alveus. During its initial course through the subjacent region (the zone of irregular cells), and even further along, the axon gives rise to several thin collaterals, some of which ascend to the plexiform subzone, where they branch repeatedly (figure 21, *i*).

3. The short-axoned cells usually display a stellate shape. Their dendrites extend in all directions, some reaching as far as the molecular layer of the fascia dentata, where they divide once. The axon of these cells may course in a number of directions, although usually with a more or less horizontal orientation, before dissolving into a large number of varicose branches that contribute to the dense intercellular plexus of the plexiform subzone.

B. Subzone of Irregular Cells

A linear array of occasional groups of well-defined cells lies just superficial to the molecular zone of the hidden part of Ammon's horn. This region contains two clear cell types.

a. One consists of pyramidal, triangular, or stellate cells with a descending axon that can be followed into the alveus. Some of their dendrites commonly enter the molecular zone of the fascia dentata (figure 21, *m*).

b. The other consists of elongated or fusiform horizontal cells with an axon that extends toward the periphery. It appears likely that these axons are the source of certain relatively thick fibers that branch repeatedly, issue horizontal collaterals to the overlying plexiform zone, and then, by an number of routes, enter the molecular layer, where they divide many times over a very broad area.

This zone may also harbor short-axoned cells with an arborization that does not extend beyond the superficial border of the pyramidal cells.

General Conclusions

1. Ammon's horn is an authentic part of the cerebral cortex that is distinguished by simplified pyramidal cell zones and a particularly complex molecular layer. Thus, the molecular layer of typical cerebral cortex is a single plexus made up of collaterals from the white matter, axonal arborizations of Golgi sensory cells (endogenous cells as well as cells with an ascending axon), and the dendritic bouquets of pyramidal cells. In contrast, the arborizations of Golgi cells in the molecular zone of Ammon's horn (which consists of the stratum radiatum, stratum lacunosum, and stratum moleculare proper) form several superimposed plexuses, each of which contacts a distinct part of the shaft and distal bouquet of the pyramidal cells.

2. Golgi sensory cells are much more abundant in Ammon's horn than in typical cerebral cortex. On the other hand, special and multipolar cells are rare or even absent in most parts of Ammon's horn.

3. The convergence of thick ascending collaterals from *regio-inferior* pyramidal cells in a horizontal band (the stratum lacunosum or lacunar layer), as well as the presence of one or more series of Golgi sensory cells in this layer, should be regarded as distinct features that serve to refine further the molecular zone.

4. The regular position of pyramidal cell bodies, and their arrangement in a single thin layer, is accompanied by an equally regular arrangement of the pericellular axonal plexuses arising from Golgi sensory cells in Ammon's horn.

5. If it is true that Golgi sensory cells (short-axoned cells) provide for associations between pyramidal cells, then it would appear that several types of association cells are found in Ammon's horn. The first type consists of cells that form associations between the somata of pyramidal cells (these include cells with a horizontal axon, as well as cells in the polymorph zone with an ascending axon). The second type consists of cells that form associations between the apical shafts of pyramidal cells (Golgi cells in the stratum radiatum).

And the third type consists of cells that form associations between the dendritic bouquets or tufts of pyramidal cells (cells in the stratum lacunosum and stratum moleculare).

Similar distinctions between sensory cells can be made quite appropriately in the fascia dentata.

The following types of Golgi association or sensory cells can be found in the latter: (1) cells that associate the distal tufts of granule cells (small Golgi cells in the molecular layer); (2) cells that contact the granule cell bodies (pyramidal cells and other cell types with an ascending axon that arborizes in the supra-granular and intergranular plexus); and (3) stellate or fusiform cells that form associations between cells in the polymorph layer.

6. Although many authors, and Schaeffer in particular, have shown on histological and embryological grounds that the fascia dentata can be regarded as cerebral cortex, it should nevertheless be considered a somewhat special type of gray matter because fibers analogous to the granule cell axon (the mossy fibers) are not found in more typical regions of the cortex.

7. Except for granule cells, all of the cell types and layers found in the fascia dentata are also found in Ammon's horn. The molecular layer of the latter simply has a very complex structure.

Chapter 5
The Olfactory Mucosa and Bulb

We shall now review what is currently known about sensory nerve endings. From the standpoint of structure-function relationships this has clearly been one of the most fertile aspects of our work. In fact, it is useful to point out early on that the sense organs almost certainly provide the best area for solving the problem of how nerve cells are connected, as well as for elucidating mechanisms underlying current transmission.

Some of the hypotheses advanced above, such as the dynamic polarization of nerve cells, have found their strongest support in the structure of the olfactory bulb and retina.

The olfactory mucosa and bulb are so intimately related that they should always be described in the same chapter on the histology of the nervous system.

The olfactory mucosa contains nerve cells that give rise to olfactory fibers that climb through the cribriform plate of the ethmoid bone to reach the brain. Thus, it constitutes a peripheral nerve center.

The olfactory bulb (which should not be referred to as the olfactory nerve because it is in fact a somewhat atrophied lobe of the cerebral cortex in humans) constitutes the terminal organ for olfactory nerve fibers. That is to say, the olfactory bulb is the site where currents from olfactory nerve fibers first influence ganglion cells in the brain.

If we compare the olfactory and retinal mechanisms, the olfactory mucosa and bulb might be viewed as two structures that are separated from one another, with the bipolar olfactory cells corresponding to the cones and rods of the retina, and the olfactory bulb corresponding to the various deeper zones of the retina (including the reticular layers, inner granular layer, ganglion cell layer, and optic nerve fibers).

The glomerular zone is the first station in the olfactory pathway since it is here that the olfactory fibers arborize, and this zone corresponds precisely to the outer reticular zone of the retina, where the first connections between cells also take place.

Olfactory Mucosa

The structure of the superior part of the nasal mucosa, which is distinguished by the fact that it contains all of the olfactory nerve cells, has been quite well known since the memorable studies of Max Schültze some time ago.

The nasal epithelium contains two principal cell types arranged in a single layer: the epithelial or support cells, and the nerve or bipolar cells.

The epithelial cells (figure 23, A, *e*) are prism shaped and display a number of indentations along their sides. These fossae are adaptations to the shape of bipolar cells, which are completely isolated from one another by the epithelial cells. At least in this regard the epithelial cells resemble Müller fibers in the retina, and it would appear that their only function is to prevent contact between nerve cells, thus preventing the horizontal spread of currents.

The bipolar or olfactory cells have an irregular, oblong, or fusiform cell body that is occupied almost entirely by the nucleus. Two processes, one outer and one inner, course through the thin protoplasmic layer that surrounds the cell bodies (figure 23, A, *f*).

The outer process is large and ends by way of several nonmotile processes at the free surface of the epithelium itself.

The inner process is very thin and varicose. As observed previously by Schültze, it displays all of the features of an axon and extends to the inferior part of the epithelium, where it then continues as an olfactory nerve fiber.

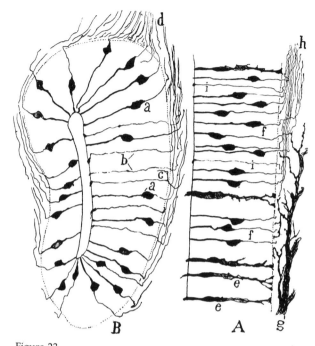

Figure 23
Bipolar olfactory cells in the rat nasal fossae (term fetus).
A: epithelium of the olfactory mucosa; *e:* epithelial cell; *f:* nerve cells; *i:* freely ending nerve fibers at the surface of the epithelium; *h:* olfactory nerve fibers; *g:* trigeminal sensory nerve.
B: a section through Jacobson's organ; *a:* bipolar cells; *b:* nerve fibers that end with a varicosity at the surface of the epithelium; *c:* a fiber that appears to arise from another fiber; *d:* descending olfactory nerve fibers.

The mucosal stroma is traversed by many bundles of olfactory fibers that are separated by a connective tissue framework and a large number of tubular glands (Bowman's glands).

Schültze suspected that the deep process of bipolar cells continues as an olfactory fiber. However, direct proof of this fact awaited the development of special analytical methods (the Ehrlich and Golgi methods). This goal has been attained only recently, thanks to studies by Arnstein, Grassi and Catronovo, van Gehuchten, and myself.

My own observations on this point demonstrate not only that one olfactory nerve fiber arises from one bipolar cell in the mucosa, but also that each fiber remains unbranched and independent during its course to the bulb, where it gives rise to a freely ending arborization. The new staining methods have not confirmed the existence of the plexuses and ramifications that several authors had described along the intra- or extraepithelial course of the olfactory fibers.

Bipolar cells are easily stained in the olfactory mucosa of mammalian embryos, particularly when my double impregnation method is employed. So also are a small number of remarkably thin fibers that course vertically through the epithelium to end by way of a conical thickening at its very surface (figure 23, A, *i*). These fibers were first noted by Brunn, who believed that I had discovered them before him. Quite recently, Lenhossék emphasized this feature, and announced that centrifugal fibers are also found in Jacobson's organ as well as in the adjacent nasal mucosa.

My own observations on this topic are in agreement with those of Brunn and Lenhossék, although they have not yet been published. Along with Lenhossék, I have observed such fibers in the nasal mucosa as well as in Jacobson's organ, although they appear to be much more common in the latter (figure 23, B, *b*). Because of their delicacy, direction, and varicose appearance, they are assimilated into the bundles of olfactory fibers. In two cases I have observed that these fibers appear to arise as branches of slightly thicker fibers coursing through the stroma of the mucosa (figure 23, B, *c*).

I am not in a position to comment on the significance of the fibers described by Brunn and Lenhossék until my ongoing work on the development of olfactory cells is completed. In any event, it might be assumed that they are sensory fibers associated with the nasal components of the ethmoidal branch of the trigeminal nerve. However, one fact does not support this presumption: trigeminal fibers destined for the nasal mucosa (inferior part) develop before the stage when the centrifugal fibers begin to stain. Furthermore, the trigeminal fibers bear no resemblance to the centrifugal fibers; the former are thick, ramify abundantly, and do not extend beyond the mucosal stroma (figure 23, B, *g*). My reservations are further substantiated by the fact that I have yet to observe Brunn fibers in newborn or very young animals.

Olfactory Bulb
The incorrectly named olfactory nerve ends above the cribriform plate of the ethmoid bone in a grayish swelling referred to as the *bulb,* into which the small nerve bundles from the nasal mucosa penetrate.

A transverse section through the bulb reveals a number of concentric layers. Starting from the surface, these include: (1) a zone of peripheral nerve fibers; (2) a zone of olfactory glomeruli; (3) a molecular zone; (4) a mitral cell zone; and (5) a zone consisting of granule cells and deep nerve fibers.

1. Superficial fiber zone   This zone consists exclusively of a large number of small olfactory fiber bundles that form a dense plexus (figure 24, D).

2. Glomerular zone   This zone is so named because at first glance the spherical or oval masses within it resemble the glomeruli of the kidney. The structure of these small organs can only be distinguished in preparations that have been stained with the silver chromate method (figure 24, A).

Golgi demonstrated as early as 1874 that two types of fibers meet in each glomerulus. One type consists of the terminal

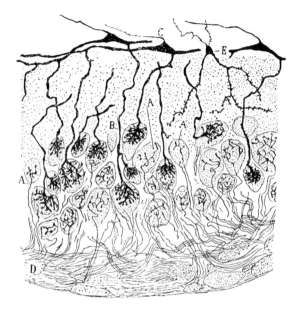

Figure 24
Dorsoventral section through the duck olfactory bulb.
A: arborizations of olfactory fibers within glomeruli; B: the descending shaft
of a large tufted cell that ends in the granule cell fringe of a glomerulus;
C: large superficial cells with a tuft (mitral cells); D: outer fiber zone; E: the
deepest granule cells.

ramifications of olfactory fibers, and the other consists of the varicose arborizations associated with the tufts or bouquets on the ends of the large dendritic shafts arising from mitral cells (in the fourth layer). According to Golgi, no functional connections are established between these two fiber types. After entering the glomerulus, the olfactory fibers ramify and form an axonal plexus, which then leaves the glomerulus by way of other centripetal nerve fibers. Because of such an arrangement, these admirable dendrites, which travel so far and ramify entirely within the glomeruli (the only region where olfactory fibers end), play not the slightest role in conduction; instead, they simply play a role in nutrition.

My own studies on the olfactory bulb in mammals, as well as studies carried out by my brother on the same organ in birds, reptiles, and amphibia, have shed light on two facts of some physiological significance that have recently been confirmed in work by van Gehuchten and Martin, Retzius, and Koelliker.

1. Olfactory fibers end freely in the glomeruli by way of varicose, thick, extremely flexuous arborizations. We have been unable to observe any terminal branches that subsequently leave the glomerular region.

2. The dendrites of mitral cells in the fourth layer, and the dendrites of certain cells in the third layer, are the only processes entering the glomeruli from the gray matter of the olfactory bulb that are in a position to gather sensory excitations. We are therefore led to assign a conductive function to these dendrites. Otherwise, sensory currents would be interrupted at the very surface of the bulb itself.

3. Molecular Layer (figures 24 and 25)   This band has a finely granular appearance and lies at the depth of the glomerular zone. Silver chromate staining reveals the presence of a few small or fusiform nerve cells that typically send a dendritic

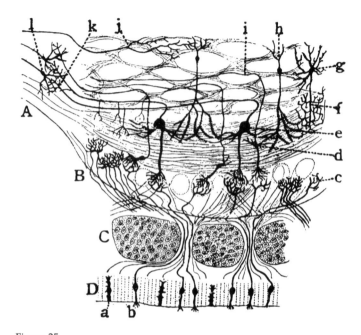

Figure 25
The mamalian olfactory system.
A: olfactory lobe; B: olfactory bulb; C: cartilage of the embryonic cribriform
plate; D: nasal mucosa; *a:* support cell; *b:* bipolar olfactory cell; *c:* arborization
of an olfactory fiber within the thickness of glomerulus; *d:* small cell with a
tuft; *e:* mitral cell; *h:* granule cells; *g:* large stellate cell with a short axon, *f,*
that ends in the molecular layer; *i:* the arborization of fibers that arise centrally.

shaft armed with a tuft or bouquet of branches to the overlying glomeruli. The deep side of the cell body issues a slender axon that bends to run caudally through the granular zone and then penetrates the bundles of myelinated axons that accumulate within the axis of the bulb.

4. Mitral Cell Layer (figures 24, C and 25, *e*)   This layer contains giant cells that may be either triangular or miter shaped, and were quite well described by Golgi. The most interesting process sprouts from the outer face of these cells, and follows a variable course through the molecular zone to end by way of an elegant varicose tuft within a glomerulus, where it comes to lie in intimate contact with the final ramifications of the olfactory fibers (figure 24, B). More or less oblique processes that ramify and disappear within the adjacent molecular zone also arise from the sides of the mitral cells. The axon is thick and arises from the inner pole of the cell. It bends shortly thereafter and follows a dorsoventral course, becoming a large fiber in the white matter of the bulb. Collaterals are issued at right angles along the final course of these axons. Such collaterals were first observed by my brother and were described in more detail by van Gehuchten and Martin; they extend toward the periphery and ramify within the thickness of the molecular zone.

5. Zone of Granule Cells and Myelinated Fibers   We are dealing here with a lattice of nerve fibers that assume a primarily dorsoventral orientation, along with islands or clusters of nerve cells. Granule cells, stellate cells, and nerve fibers may be studied in this zone.

Granule cells   These are small cells that may be either spherical, multipolar, or triangular in shape. They are so numerous that one could say that they constitute virtually the only cell type in the cell islands under consideration. They give rise to dendrites, some of which course centrally and some of which course peripherally, but they lack an axon. Based on this curious feature, they may be regarded as analogs of retinal spongioblasts (which I have termed amacrine cells because they do not have an axon).

These cells give rise to two or three very thin central processes that end a short distance away within the deep cell islands by way of thin ramifications (figures 24 E, and 25, *h*).

The peripheral process is large, and is much more substantial the closer the granule cell body is to the molecular zone. This process courses perpendicularly through the granular and mitral cell layers to enter the molecular zone, where it ends with a spine-laden tuft of divergent branches; these appear to contact the lateral dendrites of mitral cells as well as the small cells with tufted dendrites.

My brother's studies have shed light on the fact that granule cells have the same morphology and connections throughout the animal kingdom. In addition, he has shown that the peripheral process should be considered fundamental because it is never absent; on the other hand, the central processes atrophy and may even disappear as one descends the animal ladder (in amphibia and fish).

Stellate cells   These large cells were discovered by Golgi; they are few in number and are scattered irregularly throughout the granular layer. According to Golgi, the axon of these cells forms a plexus within the thickness of this layer. However, I have always observed that it ends by way of magnificent freely ending arborizations in the molecular zone (figure 25, *f*). According to van Gehuchten, there are additional types of stellate cells that are usually found at the level of the mitral cells and are characterized by extraordinarily rich dendrites.

Nerve Fibers   Almost all of the nerve fibers contributing to the small bundles that separate the islands of granule cells are simply the continuations of mitral cell axons or the axons of fusiform cells in the molecular zone. However, there are also centrifugal fibers that ramify very broadly and end freely between the granule cells, to which they probably convey some type of impulse from the brain (figure 25, *j*).

Current Pathways through the Olfactory Bulb (figure 26)
We may deduce from this summary that the transmission of olfactory impulses is not individualized; that is, transmission does not proceed from one olfactory fiber to one mitral cell, but rather from a group of olfactory fibers to a group of nerve cells. This may explain the indeterminant nature of olfactory impressions.

Based on the hypothesis that dendrites embody a receptor mechanism for currents, which the axon conducts in a cellulifugal direction, the direction of neural impulses would be as follows. An olfactory impression gathered in the mucosa by the outer process of bipolar cells is transmitted to the glomeruli by the inner process or axon. It is within the glomeruli that the dendritic tuft of the mitral cells, as well as that of the pyramidal or fusiform cells in the molecular layer, gather this impression and carry it to the brain by way of the dorsoventrally oriented axons in the granular layer. Within the brain,

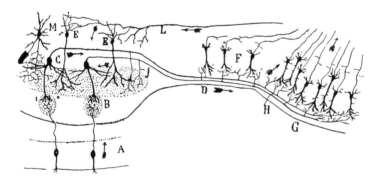

Figure 26
The course followed by neural currents through the mammalian olfactory system.
A: olfactory mucosa; B: olfactory glomerulus in the bulb; C: mitral cell; E: granule cells; D: olfactory tract; G: region of the lateral root of the olfactory nerve; F: pyramidal cells associated with the tract; M: short-axoned cell; J: mitral cell axon collaterals at the level of the olfactory bulb; H: collaterals of the same axons in the tract; I: centrifugal fiber.—The arrows indicate direction of current flow.

the terminal arborizations of these axons from the bulb deposit the impression at the level of the molecular layer of the olfactory lobe, which in turn charge the tufts or distal bouquets of pyramidal cells in this part of the cerebral cortex with the olfactory impression. In summary, the centripetal pathway for olfactory impressions has two principal branches, one in the glomeruli and the other in the cortex of the olfactory lobe. In each branch the currents become more diffused and involve a progressively larger number of nerve cells in their conduction.

The recent work of C. Calleja on the olfactory region of the mammalian brain corroborates the opinion expressed above that fibers in the *olfactory tract* end at the level of pyramidal cell bouquets in the cortex. That is, throughout their long course across the surface of the cortex, fibers in the lateral root give rise to a vast number of collaterals that ramify in the subjacent molecular layer, around the distal bouquets or tufts of pyramidal cells. No axon of a cortical cell continues on as an olfactory fiber. The essential features of this arrangement are shown diagrammatically in figure 26.

Chapter 6
The Retina

The retina is a peripheral nerve center that resembles a membranous ganglion and gives rise to most of the fibers in the optic nerve. These fibers arborize and end freely within the thickness of the geniculate bodies and superior colliculi.

The neural elements of the retina are arranged in seven layers (not counting the limiting membranes and the pigmented zone):

1. The rods and cones
2. The outer granule cells, or visual cell bodies
3. The outer plexiform or molecular layer
4. The inner granule cells
5. The inner plexiform or molecular layer
6. The ganglion cells
7. The fibers of the optic nerve

All of these elements are both supported and isolated by large cells that stretch from front to back, that is, from the outer face of the retina to the zone containing rods and cones. These cells have been called Müller fibers, or retinal epithelial cells. Like the supporting cells of the olfactory mucosa, the sides of Müller fibers bear vast numbers of fossae or indentations that serve as receptacles for retinal cells and nerve fibers. The nuclei of Müller fibers are found at the level of the inner granular layer, and each end of the cytoplasm or cell body condenses to form part of a homogenous limiting membrane, one below the cones and rods, and the other on the ventral surface of the retina (figure 27, *t*). The Müller fibers are completely independent since they form nothing but simple con-

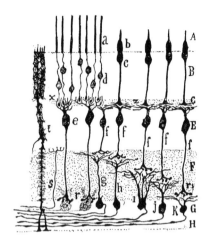

Figure 27
A transverse section through the mammalian retina.
A: layer of cones and rods; B: visual cell bodies (outer granule cells); C: outer plexiform layer; E: bipolar cell layer (inner granule cells); F: inner plexiform layer; G: ganglion cell layer; H: optic nerve fiber layer; *a*: rod; *b*: cone; *c*: cone cell body; *d*: rod cell body; *e*: bipolar cell associated with a rod; *f*: bipolar cells associated with cones; *g, h, i, j, k*: ganglion cells that ramify in different levels of the inner plexiform zone; *r*: inner arborization of rod bipolar cells that form connections with the ganglion cells; *r*: inner arborization of cone bipolar cells; *t*: Müller or epithelial cell; *x*: contacts between rods and their bipolar cells; *z*: contacts between the cones and their bipolar cells; *s*: centrifugal nerve fiber.

tacts between themselves, or with the neural elements that they support.

It seems quite likely that Müller fibers play a role isolating neural currents in view of the fact that they are absent only in those zones of the retina where fiber connections are established, that is, where currents pass.

1. Layer of Rods and Cones (figure 27, A)
We shall not deal here with the very unusual physical and chemical properties of these organelles because they are quite well known thanks to the work of Müller, Schültze, Krause, Koelliker, Hoffmann, Ranvier, Boll, Kühn, and others. Instead,

I shall focus entirely on the morphological properties that have shaped our point of view.

The rod (figure 27, *a*) is a thin fiber in mammals and nocturnal birds, and is quite thick in amphibians, diurnal birds, and fish; it is entirely absent in reptiles.

The cone is the only type of fiber in the reptilian retina. It is quite abundant in diurnal birds, rare in nocturnal birds, and much less frequent than rods in the mammalian retina, except in the central fossa, which we know contains only cones. As illustrated in figure 27, *b*, the mammalian cone is a large, bottle-shaped process that is shorter than the rods. From the histogenetic point of view, cones and rods are not complete cells. They are rather a secretion product of cells in the subjacent layer (the outer granule cells) that are highly differentiated in terms of fine structural details. They can be thought of as forming a remarkably reinforced epithelial layer.

2. Layer of Visual Cell Bodies (figure 27, B)
The visual cell bodies, which are also known as outer granule cells, represent the untransformed living cytoplasm of cones and rods. Therefore, they are continuous with the cones and rods across the external limiting membrane, which produces a large number of rounded indentations on the cells. It is necessary in the following description to distinguish between cell bodies that give rise to a cone or to a rod.

The cone cell body (figure 27, *c*) lies near the outer limiting membrane and has a large oval nucleus. The bottom or inner part of the cell body cytoplasm continues as a straight fiber that gives rise to a conic dilation (the foot of the cone), after entering the outer plexiform zone. Several freely ending, horizontally oriented fibers arise from the base of this conic dilation.

The rod cell body (figure 27, *d*) may lie at various depths within the outer granular layer. The oval nucleus of rods is smaller than that of the cones, and the cytoplasm gives rise to two fibers, one ascending and the other descending. The ascending process is thin and varicose and ends as a rod, whereas the descending process, which is also very thin, enters the outer plexiform zone, where it ends freely in a tiny sphere with no branches.

The processes that earlier researchers, as well as certain contemporary scientists such as Tartuferi and Dogiel, have described as arising from the terminal sphere of rods are due either to biases associated with certain schools of thought or to simple illusions; nothing of this sort has been observed with the methods of Golgi and Ehrlich.

I mention biases associated with schools of thought because during the anastomosis era it would have been truly heretical to assume that cells like rods, which play such an important role in the phenomenon of vision, could remain isolated, i.e., without establishing continuity with the innumerable fibers thought to exist in the outer plexiform zone. Happily, the truth now reveals a way out of this dilemma. As we shall soon see, the doctrine of transmission by contact implies that the activity produced in rods can be gathered by certain bipolar cells and conveyed individually to certain nerve centers.

Outer Plexiform Layer (figure 27, C and 28, I)
Many dendrites from cells in the subjacent layer (the inner granule cell layer), as well as a large number of basilar fibers from the cone feet, intermingle in the outer plexiform layer.

This zone should be subdivided into superior and inferior levels, each associated with the connections of one type of nerve cell.

The superior level (figure 27, x) is a region where the terminal rod spherules meet and contact the tufts or ascending bouquets of certain bipolar cells that are associated with rods. The inferior level (figure 27, z) is a region where the feet and basilar processes of cones aggregate to contact the ascending, flattened processes of certain bipolar cells that are associated with cones.

Inner Granule Cell Layer (figure 27, E)
This is the most complex layer in the retina. For descriptive purposes it should be divided into three subzones that contain

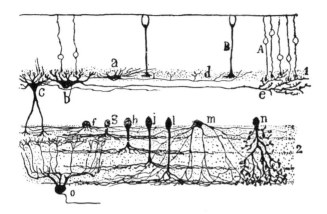

Figure 28
Transverse section through a mammalian retina.
A: Outer granule cells or rod cell bodies; B: cone cell bodies; *a*: outer or small horizontal cell; *b*: inner or large horizontal cell; *c*: inner horizontal cell with descending dendritic processes; *e*: flattened arborization of one of these large cells; *f*, *g*, *h*, *j*, *l*: spongioblasts that ramify within various levels of the inner plexiform zone; *m*, *n*: diffuse spongioblasts; *o*: bistratified ganglion cell; 1: outer plexiform zone; 2: inner plexiform zone.

(1) horizontal cells (which have been referred to as subreticular cells, stellate cells, and so on), (2) bipolar cells, and (3) spongioblasts.

Horizontal Cells   These cells have been examined in almost every number of the vertebrate series by Krause and Schiefferdecker, although a proper understanding of their role emerged from the work of Tartuferi, Dogiel, and myself.

There are two major types of horizontal cells in mammals, the small or outer horizontal cells and the large or inner horizontal cells, as well as several less important varieties. The small horizontal cells (figure 28, *a*) are flat and stellate shaped, and lie immediately adjacent to the outer plexiform zone. The many divergent, branching processes that sprout from their periphery form an extremely dense plexus below the feet of the cones. The axon of these cells (figure 28, *d*) is thin and courses horizontally for variable distances before entering the inner granule cell zone, where it ends by giving rise to several terminal branches. Along its course, the axon emits a number of ramified, freely ending collaterals.

The large horizontal cells (figure 28, *b*) usually lie internal to the small horizontal cells, and are distinguished from them on the basis of size.

They have thick, horizontally oriented dendrites that are rather short, and end in short, fingerlike, ascending branches. The neural process or axon is large and horizontally oriented, and was first observed by Tartuferi. They have recently been stained with methylene blue by Dogiel, who assumed that they course horizontally for a variable distance before descending abruptly through the various layers of the retina and contributing fibers to the optic nerve. In my opinion, however, the Russian scholar [Dogiel] fell victim to an illusion arising from the difficulty of establishing the entire course of nerve fibers from cells in particular layers of retinal whole mounts stained with this reagent.

My own recent observations, which have been carried out on large horizontal sections of the retina with the double silver chromate method, indicate that these axons never descend, and thus never leave the outer plexiform zone; instead, they end in this zone by way of an enormously broad, varicose arborization after following a very long course. Each fiber of this ramification extends a short branch that ends in a varicosity near the level of the rod spherules (figure 28, *e*).

My most recent discovery is that these axonal arborizations are found in sparrows as well. They are less extensive here than in mammals, although the branches, which also issue thin ascending spines, are more densely packed. These arborizations have been shown to be even smaller and simpler in gallinaceae, although I have not been able to confirm whether they correspond precisely to the arborizations in sparrows mentioned above.

We should also mention one variety of large or inner horizontal cell that is similar to others in this class but in addition is characterized by the presence of one or two dendrites that descend to ramify in the inner plexiform zone (figure 28, *c*). Tartuferi and Dogiel believe that all of the large horizontal cells give rise to descending processes, although my own studies leave no doubt about the existence of cells in this category with no descending dendrites.

Bipolar Cells   Tartuferi and Dogiel demonstrated that these cells are fusiform and give rise to two processes, one ascending and the other descending. There is always one descending process that ends as a flattened tuft at various levels of the inner plexiform zone. The ascending process is often branched and gives rise to an abundant ramification that becomes horizontally oriented within inner parts of the outer plexiform zone (figure 27, *e*, *f*).

The following observations from my own work may be added to the descriptions provided by these authors.

1. The tuft formed by the ascending process, as well as by the varicose branches, ends freely. Therefore, the anastomoses that these authors described in the plexus where the processes ramify, do not exist. These descriptions were influenced by the scientific milieu at the time.

2. All bipolar cells are not identical, since they differ in shape and size. The major types include the following. (1) Some bipolar cells have a thin, ascending tuft that ends freely among the rod spherules (figure 27, *e*). Because the location of these spherules is so precisely correlated with the fibers of this terminal tuft, and because no other cellular processes reach this level, we are left with the conclusion that these bipolar cells are in a position to gather the specific activity generated by rods. Based on this, I have called them rod bipolar cells. (2) A second type of bipolar cell gives rise to a flattened tuft that ramifies in the second level of the outer plexiform zone, where the basal fiber of the cones ramifies (figure 27, *f*). This special correspondence has led me to designate such cells as cone bipolar cells. In view of the disposition of their outer tufts, they can only contact cones. (3) Some

bipolar cells are related to cones as well as to rods. They have a very large ascending tuft that covers an area of the retina equal to that established by the small horizontal cell. The branches of this outer bouquet are oriented horizontally and ramify many times. They occasionally give rise to ascending collateral spines that contact rod spherules, while others display the appearance of cone bipolar cell branches.

3. The inner tuft of most if not all of the rod bipolar cells makes contact with cell bodies in the ganglion cell layer, while the descending tuft of cone bipolar cells, and perhaps of the giant bipolar cells, ends in any one of the five arborization levels that essentially form the inner plexiform zone (figure 27, *r*, *s*).

Spongioblasts (figure 28, *f*, *g*, *h*, and so on)
The spongioblasts lie within the deepest part of the inner granular zone, and all of their processes are directed toward the inner plexiform zone, where they ramify and end. Several authors are of the opinion that they form horizontally oriented plexuses in this region.

My own observations on these unique cells, which, as Dogiel pointed out, lack an axon, have allowed me to confirm the following observations.

1. Each of the five arborization zones in the inner plexiform zone is associated with its own type of spongioblast. That is to say, five types of spongioblasts can be distinguished on the basis of the level of the inner plexiform zone to which they send their terminal arborization. Therefore, some spongioblasts give rise to a shaft (or to several shafts) that ramifies in the first level; other spongioblasts have a process that ramifies in the second level, and so on (figure 28, *f*, *g*, *h*).

2. In addition to spongioblasts with processes that ramify entirely within one level of the inner plexiform layer, and may thus be considered stratified, there are spongioblasts with processes that spread throughout most of the thickness of the inner plexiform zone. These cells might be called diffuse spongioblasts (figure 28, *m*, *n*). It is important to note, however,

that a majority of the branches of these diffuse spongioblasts are clustered in the innermost level of the inner plexiform zone.

3. Spongioblasts form at least two kinds of flattened arborizations within each level of the inner plexiform zone. Some arborizations are very broadly distributed and consist of thin, horizontally oriented fibers that course in many directions with the appearance of axons, while others are much more restricted, less dense, and more irregular; the latter consist of thick, flexuous fibers that ramify many times. These arborizations are frequently intermingled with others that are characterized by thick fibers with spiny horizontal branches, particularly in levels two, three, and four.

4. In addition to extensive spongioblast arborizations, each level of the inner plexiform zone contains broad, horizontally oriented ramifications that are formed by the dendrites of ganglion cells in the sixth layer. These dendrites are concentrated in the lower part of each level.

In summary, each level appears to consist of an outer plane that is formed by spongioblast branches, an inner plane that contains the arborizations of unistratified ganglion cells, and a middle plane where the inner tufts of cone bipolar cells are aligned along, perhaps, with the tufts of certain rod bipolar cells, although this remains to be proven. These three fiber plexuses are not entirely segregated because branches from each climb or descend at different points, intermingling and forming a very dense feltwork.

I have set the number of horizontal plexuses in the mammalian retina at five. Of these, the first, second, fourth, and fifth are much thicker and more obvious than the third. It goes without saying that this number should not be considered absolute, as further work may reveal additional levels. This is particularly likely considering the nature of the retina in birds and reptiles; there the inner plexiform zone is more fully developed, and we have been able to distinguish seven levels or concentric fiber plexuses in the thickest part of this membrane, although only five are well developed and contain rich arborizations.

Inner Plexiform Layer (figures 27, F and 28, 2)
We have already described the major features of this retinal zone in the previous section. Three cell types contact one another in the inner plexiform layer: spongioblasts, bipolar cells, and ganglion cells. Furthermore, in mammals, this layer contains a small number of horizontal spongioblasts with branches that disappear within one of the various levels described above.

In order to assure a large number of contact points and to avoid communication that might compromise transmission through specific pathways, nature has provided certain zones or concentric levels for the establishment of particular types of contacts. Animals with smaller and more numerous bipolar cells have a thicker inner plexiform layer with more levels.

Ganglion Cell Layer (figure 27, G).
It is well known that the axon of these cells continues as a fiber in the optic nerve. The cell body is oval, piriform, or crescent shaped, while the dendrites arise from its outer face and ramify as horizontally oriented plexuses at various depths of the inner plexiform layer. All ganglion cells may be assigned to one of three classes on the basis of how their outer dendritic process arborizes.

1. Unistratified cells (figure 27, g, h, i, j, k) give rise to a dendrite that ramifies within a single level of the inner plexiform zone. Because there are five such levels, it follows that some cells arborize within the first level, others send their processes to the second level, and so on.

2. Multistratified cells (figure 28, *o*) have a dendrite that forms two or more concentric plexuses within exactly corresponding levels of the inner plexiform layer.

3. Diffuse cells have a loosely organized, ascending arborization that is unstratified and extends throughout most of the thickness of the inner plexiform layer.

Ganglion cells may also be classified according to size into small, medium, and giant cells. Although there are exceptions, we maintain that smaller cells have smaller terminal ramifications that arborize in more inferior levels of the inner plexiform layer.

Optic Nerve Fiber Layer (figure 27, H)
The majority of axons in this zone are the simple continuations of the basal or functional process of ganglion cells. However, some of these axons should be regarded as centrifugal fibers that arise in optic centers of the brain. I discovered these fibers in the avian retina, and Monakow inferred their existence on the basis of studies in pathological material (figure 27, *s*).

Course of Light-Induced Impulses in the Retina
From what has just been discussed, nothing could be easier than following the course taken by impressions gathered by the rods and cones. However, since the connections of rods and cones are different, and since it is quite likely that each type of visual cell is influenced by a distinct quality of light (rods by colorless luminous intensity, and cones by color), it is convenient to consider separately the route taken by impressions received by each type of visual cell.

Impression Received by Rods   The impression is first carried to the outer plexiform zone; there it is transferred to the ascending tuft of rod bipolar cells, which transmit the impression directly to the perikaryon of giant ganglion cells. The activity is then transmitted along axons of the optic fiber layer, optic nerves, and optic tracts to end on the peripheral dendritic tufts of certain nerve cells in the geniculate bodies or colliculi.

I discovered how optic nerve fibers end during the course of my studies on the avian optic lobe. Here, each fiber gives rise to a magnificent, freely ending arborization that contacts the dendrites of various types of fusiform cells.

P. Ramón also demonstrated that mammalian optic fibers give rise to freely ending arborizations among the dendritic

ramifications of large stellate and fusiform cells in the geniculate bodies as well as in the superior colliculi (figure 29, C).
And, finally, van Gehuchten has quite recently described the
same type of endings in the optic lobe of the chick, as well as
the intermingling of axons and dendrites that occurs in the
superficial layers of this organ.

Impression Received by Cones   Such activity is conducted immediately to the deep level of the outer reticular zone, where
it is gathered by the thick tufts of cone bipolar cells and directed to one of the five levels of the inner plexiform zone
(depending on which type of cone bipolar cell is involved),
where it in turn reaches the dendritic tufts of ganglion cells.
Finally, ganglion cell axons are responsible for the ultimate
conduction of currents to optic centers in the brain. It is not
yet clear whether there is a special region of the brain devoted
to storing these impressions.

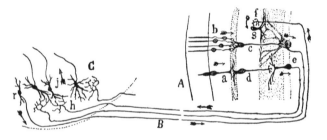

Figure 29
The path taken by neural activity from cones and rods to the geniculate body
A: retina; B: optic nerve; C: geniculate body; *a*: cone; *b*: rod; *d*: cone bipolar
cell; *c*: rod bipolar cell; *e*: ganglion cell; *f*: centrifugal nerve fiber; *g*: spongioblast; *h*: freely ending arborizations of fibers from the retina; *j*: nerve cell with
a dendritic bouquet whose function is to gather activity from optic fibers; *r*:
probable cells of origin for the centrifugal fibers.—Arrows indicate the direction of current flow.

Several important consequences follow from the organization of retinal and central visual pathways.

1. Activity associated with visual cells is always gathered by dendrites, transmitted by axons, and distributed by the arborizations of nerve fibers. That is, cells in the retina, like those in the olfactory bulb and all other centers where the direction of current flow is obvious, display one mechanism for receiving currents (cell bodies and dendrites) and another for conducting and distributing these currents.

2. Activity in the retina is not transmitted through isolated, longitudinally oriented series of elements, but rather through a group of cells with interconnections such that, as the activity progresses through the retina, more cells are involved in its conduction. For example, activity transmitted by a cone is gathered by the flattened tufts of several bipolar cells. Since these bipolar cells give rise to descending processes that end in various levels of the inner plexiform layer, it follows that a substantial number of ganglion cells (more, in any event, than the number of bipolar cells involved) also participate in conducting the activity. Finally, each fiber in the optic tract contacts many ganglion cells in the optic centers by way of its extensive, freely ending arborizations. On the other hand, conduction is much less divergent and more precise at the level of the central fossa of the retina. In this region, it would appear that each cone foot is in contact with the tuft of one bipolar cell, and the descending process of this bipolar cell is in contact with a limited part of the dendritic arborization of the ganglion cell. This pattern of arborization, combined with the extremely delicate structure of cones and the other elements involved in this conduction pathway, is sufficient to explain the very high level of visual acuity associated with the central fossa of the retina.

3. Horizontal cells appear to be involved in forming associations between two areas of the retina that are separated by variable distances. The elements that appear to be associated are cones and rods.

4. Spongioblasts appear to lie outside the chain of retinal nerve cells; nothing is known about their function in view of the fact that they lack an axon, and their one process involves contact with ganglion cells. We might, however, suggest that because spongioblasts are the only elements of the retina to receive terminal arborizations from centrifugal fibers, they may serve to carry some type of activity from the brain to ganglion cells, impulses that may be necessary for the functional interplay of bipolar cell connections. In any event, the role played by spongioblasts must be quite important because they are present in all vertebrates, and because their numbers and types increase either along the edge of the *fovea* in a great many animals (reptiles and birds), or in neighboring regions (mammals). Furthermore, a very complex system of spongioblasts is found in the thickest and most highly refined retinas, such as those found in birds and reptiles.[1]

---

1. My fundamental ideas on the structure of the retina have been accepted by Retzius, His, and van Gehuchten, whose latest studies include diagrams very similar to my own.

Chapter 7

Nerve Endings of the Inner Ear

The Swedish scholar G. Retzius made use of the silver chromate double-staining method that I had developed to resolve at last the difficult problem of how fibers of the auditory nerve end in both the organ of Corti (in the cochlea) and the epithelium of the cristae acusticae (in the semicircular canals). In doing so, he left no doubt that these fibers give rise to freely ending, intercellular ramifications, which are not continuous with the ciliated cells that have been described in the epithelia.

In fact, Retzius knew that the terminal fibers of the auditory nerve are comparable in every way to those of the olfactory nerve since both represent the distal processes of bipolar cells. The only difference between them is the location of the cell bodies of origin. As we have already seen, in the olfactory mucosa the cells are found in the middle of the epithelium and the distal process is short and unramified. On the other hand, the auditory bipolar cell is located some distance from the epithelium (in the ganglia along the course of nerve branches from the cochlea and semicircular canals) and its distal process gives rise to many ascending branches that end among the epithelial cells. Thus, the auditory epithelial cells, which are equipped with cilia, are somewhat equivalent to the rods and cones of the retina since they form an intermediate epithelial link between an external agent (sound waves) and receptor nerve fibers.

My own recent studies fully confirm Retzius' description. A section through a semicircular canal from a rat fetus at term is presented in figure 30. Nerve fibers from bipolar cells residing far from the epithelium can be seen to penetrate the crista

acustica, which has been cut transversely; the terminal ramifications are varicose and form small arcs (directed toward the
epithelium) at their point of origin; the branches end in a
varicosity near the free surface of the epithelium. This figure
also shows other nerve endings of the same type in other parts
of the epithelium outside the region of the cristae acusticae. I
have not been able to determine the nature of these endings,
although it seems likely that they are also fibers associated
with the auditory nerve (figure 30, D).

From what has just been said, it is fair to conclude that the
mode of auditory nerve endings lends further support to the

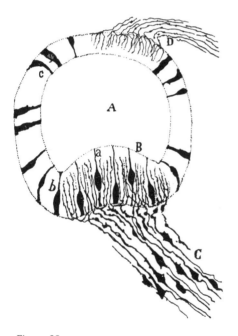

Figure 30
A transverse section through the crista acustica of a semicircular canal of a rat
fetus.
A: semicircular canal; B: crista acustica; C: bundle of nerve fibers arising from
bipolar cells; D: small bundle of nerve fibers ending in the superior part of
the semicircular canal; *a:* bipolar epithelial cell; *b* and *c:* epithelial cell types.

hypothesis of the dynamic polarization of nerve cells, which has already been mentioned a number of times. The outer process of bipolar auditory cells is thicker than the inner process and may be regarded as a dendrite, while the inner or deep process is much thinner, and may be considered a true axon. The stimulus gathered by epithelial cells is conveyed to the dendritic ramifications, and then to the perikaryon and its nerve fiber. The excitation is then conducted by the nerve fiber to the brain stem, where it is clear that auditory nerve terminal arborizations intermingle and make contact with another series of nerve cells.

In a recent study (*Die Nervenendigungen in der Maculae und Cristae acusticae*, 1893), Lenhossék has presented a description of the auditory endings that differs somewhat from my own. According to Lenhossék, auditory fibers penetrate the thickness of the epithelium and dissolve into freely ending arborizations that lie below the deep end of the ciliated cells. This implies that there are two types of ramifications, one arising below the epithelium, which I had described, and another, not present in my preparations, lying within the thickness of the epithelium below the ciliated cells. The differences between our descriptions are probably due to the fact that we did not study the same stage of development. Lenhossék dealt with rats that were several days old, whereas I used very young fetuses of the same animal where it was quite likely that the secondary, final ramifications had not yet developed. Nevertheless, Retzius, van Gehuchten, von Lenhossék, and I all agree on two fundamental points: freely ending interepithelial arborizations, and contacts between nerve fibers and ciliated cells.

Chapter 8
Neural Ganglia

Ganglia may be divided into three types based on their structure and physiology: cerebrospinal, sympathetic chain, and visceral.

Cerebrospinal Ganglia

Work by Ranvier, Lenhossék, Retzius, and others established some time ago that spinal ganglia (figures 31 and 34, D, *j*) are formed by piriform cells with a single short process that divides into two nerve fibers; one is relatively thin and continues on as a fiber in the dorsal or sensory root of the spinal cord, while the other is thicker and courses peripherally to join the associated spinal nerve, where it mingles with motor fibers arising in the ventral horn of the spinal cord. If the peripheral fiber could be followed over a sufficient distance it would be found to end in either a Pacinian or Meissner cell or on an epithelial surface, although such endings always end freely in a swelling.

It has been known since the work of Lenhossék that each ganglion cell is surrounded by an endothelial capsule. Inside this capsule, that is, between the capsule and the cytoplasm of the ganglion cell, lies the pericellular arborization of a nerve fiber whose origin is unknown. These arborizations were first described in the frog by Ehrlich, and I subsequently demonstrated them in mammals. These arborizations prove that a ganglion cell may receive impulses from other cells, in addition to transmitting current from the periphery to the spinal cord. From the results of some of my own studies, it would appear

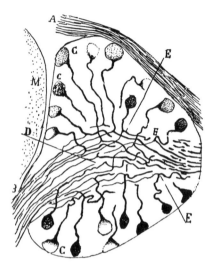

Figure 31
Section of a spinal ganglion from an eight-day-old rat.
A: ventral root; B: dorsal root; C: ganglion cell bodies; D: medial or central fibers that arise from the branch point, E, of the single process of ganglion cells; M: spinal cord.

that these plexuses may arise from cells in the great sympathetic chain.

In fact, nerve fibers from sympathetic ganglia can be followed into their accompanying rami communicantes and then into spinal ganglia. Such fibers are thick in vertebrates, and branch at least three times after penetrating the spinal ganglion. A number of these branches seem to disappear within the thickness of the ganglion and may give rise to pericellular arborizations. In addition, other sympathetic processes enter the ventral root, thus gaining access to the spinal cord, where they may end freely. This is speculation rather than demonstrated fact, however, since I have not been able to follow sympathetic fibers in the ventral root all the way to the spinal cord.

All of the ganglia that lie along the course of the cranial nerves, including the vagus, glossopharyngeal, facial, and trigeminal nerves, have the same structure.

Sympathetic Chain Ganglia

It had been thought for a number of years that all of the processes of multipolar sympathetic neurons were axonal in nature, and that they continued on as fibers of Remak.

However, the dissociation method used by Ranvier and others to examine the morphology of these elements is seriously flawed because cellular processes are broken and deformed, thus rendering it impossible to follow them as far as their terminal branches. About four years ago (November 1889), Koelliker used the rapid Golgi method to resolve this problem in a definitive way, looking specifically at the cervical ganglia of the sympathetic chain in the cow. First, he confirmed the classical view that sympathetic cells are multipolar and followed the processes over considerable distances, observing that they ramify many times and end by branching. It appeared to him that a number of these cellular processes continue on as fibers of Remak, although he no doubt would have considered others that ramify extensively as a separate category. However, instead of categorically stating that the latter end freely, he was inclined to presume that they anastomose with bundles of Remak fibers from certain sympathetic cells.

The wave of confirmations generated by Koelliker's work, as well as the obvious importance of the problem, prompts me to include the results of a number of our studies on sympathetic ganglia of the chick embryo (figures 32 and 34) that establish several important anatomical features.

1. Sympathetic cells are multipolar and give rise to axons as well as to a large number of short processes that end freely within the thickness of the ganglia themselves.

2. The longitudinal commissure, which forms part of the great sympathetic chain, is made up of axons from cells in each of the ganglia that give rise to varicose, freely ending

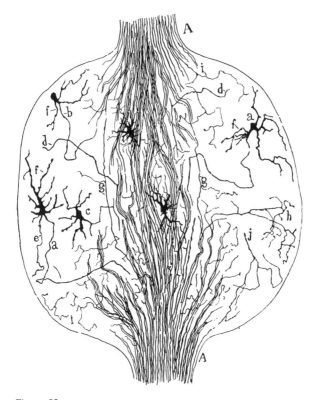

Figure 32
Longitudinal section of a thoracic sympathetic ganglion from a chick embryo
on the fifteenth day of incubation.
A: longitudinal trunk of the sympathetic chain with sympathetic ganglia along
its course; a: sympathetic cell with an axon entering the longitudinal trunk; b:
a smaller cell of the same type; e, f: dendrites of sympathetic cells; g: collaterals
of fibers in the longitudinal bundle; h, i, j: freely ending nerve fibers in the
ganglion.

arborizations surrounding the perikarya and short processes of ganglion cells. The longitudinal trunk also contains myelinated fibers. Many authors have observed that a large proportion of these fibers arise from the ventral roots.

3. Centrifugal fibers from the spinal cord also course through the ventral roots to enter the thickness of each ganglion, where they give rise to freely ending arborizations.

4. Commissural, longitudinal, or interganglionic fibers occasionally give rise to collaterals that enable sympathetic cells to establish relationships with a great many cells in neighboring ganglia, and so on. These collaterals are rare and difficult to stain in mammals, possibly explaining why Fusari failed to observe them in the ganglia of dogs and cats. They are, however, a constant feature of chick embryos.

I had not been able to establish with certainty the number of processes arising from individual cells in my material, although I was inclined to suggest that there are one or more, depending on the volume of the cell.

However, later definitive preparations of adult mammalian ganglia persuaded me to conclude that sympathetic cells, like those in the cerebrospinal ganglia, give rise to a single axon (figure 33, C) that continues as a fiber of Remak and enters one of the longitudinal bundles associated with each ganglion, or courses through one of the visceral nerves to the visceral organs. The view that the central nervous system establishes relationships with cells in the ganglia of the sympathetic chain has been fully confirmed by the latest work of Retzius, van Gehuchten, and L. Sala.

I have also been able to establish several additional features in recent unpublished work on the sympathetic chain in 14- to 18-day-old chick embryos, as well as in the rat embryo and the newborn mouse.

a. The rami communicantes contain two fiber types in birds as well as in mammals. One type consists of sympathetic fibers that represent the axons of sympathetic cells in the corresponding ganglion. Each pair of rami communicantes sends one bundle of Remak fibers to the ventral branch of a spinal

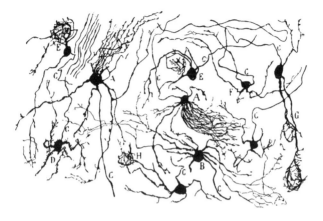

Figure 33
Different types of sympathetic cells in the superior and inferior ganglia of the adult dog.
A: cell with a dense tuft of short processes; B: another cell with short, thin processes that ramify extensively; D: cell with a small number of short, hairlike processes; F: cell with a very small number of short, fine processes; G: cell with two processes that ramify around two neighboring elements; C: ganglion cell axons.

nerve and another bundle of Remak fibers to the dorsal branch. After entering these branches, the Remak fibers course toward the periphery along with the motor and sensory nerve fibers. This arrangement had been alluded to by several authors, although definite proof was lacking. Fortunately, I have been able to demonstrate in a large number of perfectly stained preparations that this is indeed the case, and thus have been able to observe the sympathetic cell of origin, its axon, and the continuation of this process through the rami communicantes and over rather long distances through both the ventral and dorsal rami of each spinal nerve.

The second type consists of a smaller number of myelinated fibers that are associated with the ventral and dorsal roots. Upon entering the sympathetic ganglion, many of these fibers curve to penetrate the longitudinal commissure. I have not been able to determine precisely the nature of these fibers

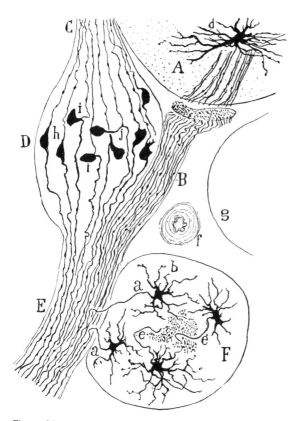

Figure 34

Spinal and sympathetic ganglia in the cervical region of a chick embryo on the seventeenth day of incubation.

A: spinal cord with one ventral root cell (*d*); B: ventral or motor root; C: dorsal or sensory root; D: spinal ganglion; E: cervical spinal nerve; F: sympathetic ganglion; *a:* sympathetic axons forming the rami communicantes and coursing toward the accompanying spinal nerve; *b:* dendrites of sympathetic cells; *e:* sympathetic axons that course horizontally to enter the longitudinal commissure of the ganglion; *h:* fusiform spinal ganglion cells; *i:* transition of a bipolar cell to a unipolar cell in the spinal ganglion; *j:* frankly unipolar cell; *f:* cross section of an artery; *g:* body of a cervical vertebra.

because their extraordinary course makes it impossible to follow them from beginning to end in any one section. Nevertheless, I have observed that some fibers in the ventral root are shorter and give rise to freely ending arborizations that end among the cells of sympathetic ganglia.

   b. In addition to medium-sized sympathetic fibers destined for the ventral and dorsal rami of the spinal nerves, each pair of rami communicantes in the mammal contains thicker sympathetic fibers that behave somewhat differently. These fibers bifurcate as they enter the spinal nerve; one branch continues through the dorsal or ventral ramus, while the other, which may consist of a pair, enters the ventral root and appears to course towards the spinal cord. I have even observed one very thick sympathetic fiber that gave rise to seven branches as it entered the spinal nerve; two small branches entered the ventral ramus, one entered the dorsal ramus, one passed through the spinal ganglion and appeared to continue on through the dorsal root, and three entered the ventral root and coursed towards the spinal cord.

   It seems very likely that branches from the bifurcation of sympathetic cells, or large axon collaterals from these cells, enter the spinal cord. However, it is not clear to me whether these branches give rise to pericellular plexuses around unipolar elements in the spinal ganglia.

Visceral Ganglia

The sympathetic system also includes the ganglia of the celiac plexus (semilunar and solar) and hypogastric plexus, as well as the ophthalmic, the sphenopalatine, and probably the cardiac ganglia. As we have just seen, cells in these ganglia give rise to two classes of process: *dendritic ramifications* and the *axon* or *fiber of Remak,* which leaves the ganglion and usually enters the longitudinal sympathetic commissure or the rami communicantes.

   Nevertheless, there are two types of ganglia that are poorly understood. The morphology of these ganglia is not known, and thus it is unclear whether they follow the sympathetic pattern or have unique characteristics. One type of ganglion is found in the intestine (Auerbach's and Meissner's plexuses), bladder, and esophagus, while the other consists of monocellular ganglia within glandular tissues or within the thickness of the villi. The latter include interstitial cells in the crypts of Lieberkühn, in the pancreas, in the salivary glands, and elsewhere.

To avoid paraphrasing, I shall refer to the latter as interstitial ganglia and the former as visceral ganglia proper.

Visceral Ganglia Proper
These may be considered the ganglia in Auerbach's and Meissner's plexuses. For the sake of clarity and convenience, I shall restrict the following description to Meissner's plexus in view of the fact that the ganglia in both plexuses are structurally analogous.

It is common knowledge that Meissner's plexus (figure 35, C and *c*) lies below the crypts of Lieberkühn in the submucosal connective tissue and that it presents two elements for examination: fasciculi of nerve fibers and ganglia.

Fasciculi (figure 36)   Most of what is known about these fasciculi has come from researchers using the acid-gold chloride method, as well as from E. Müller and Berkley, who applied the silver chromate method to this problem. Thus, I shall only briefly review this work to avoid repeating information that is only too well known.

Each small bundle contains a variable number of well separated, varicose nerve fibers that vary in thickness, lack myelin, and are held together along their length by a cement that is not stained by silver chromate, even in the most successful preparations. Chiasmas are formed in regions where several bundles meet. E. Müller noted that each nerve fiber remains completely separate at the level of these intersections, while passing from one fascicle to another on the same or on the opposite side of the chiasma (figure 36, B, *g*). Some of the

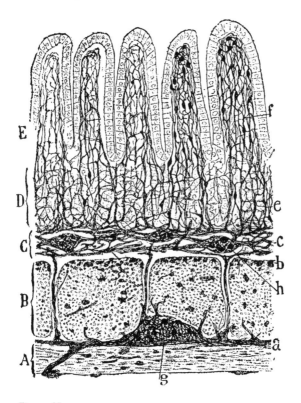

Figure 35
Longitudinal section through the small intestine of the guinea pig. This semi-diagrammatic drawing is designed to show all of the plexuses and ganglia of the intestine.
A: Longitudinal muscle fiber layer; B: circular muscle fiber layer; C: submucosal connective tissue with Meissner's plexus and ganglia; D: layer of crypts of Lieberkühn; E: villi; *a:* Auerbach's plexus; *g:* Auerbach's ganglion; *b:* cross section of a deep muscle plexus; *c:* fasciculi of Meissner's plexus; *e:* bundles of the periglandular plexus; *f:* intravillous plexus.

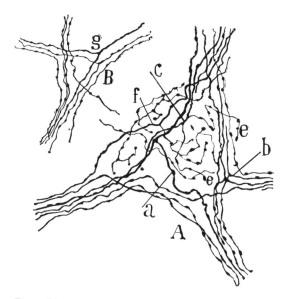

Figure 36
A: Meissner's ganglion in the guinea pig (the cells were not stained); *a:* large bifurcating fiber; *b:* smaller bifurcating fiber; *c:* fiber of passage giving rise to two collaterals; *e:* free ending of a collateral; *f:* another fiber of passage giving rise to a collateral.
B: Meissner's plexus chiasma; *g:* nerve fiber bifurcation.

thick nerve fibers bifurcate, and the branches, which may or may not be of equal diameter, then enter two distinct fasciculi.

Ganglia (figures 36, A; 37; and 39)   A great deal of the material that I have examined is from the guinea pig, where the ganglia are made up of the following components: two to eight nerve cells, fibers passing through, and collaterals.

   a. Cells (figure 37) Although they are usually rather large, the size of these cells is variable. Several authors, including Schwalbe, Ranvier, Toldt, and others, have noted that they are distinctly multipolar or stellate in outline, and give rise to

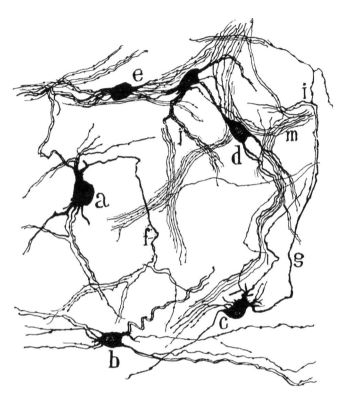

Figure 37
Meissner ganglion cells in the guinea pig (The ganglia themselves are not shown).

a, b, c: individually stained multipolar cells; some of their processes can be followed over relatively long distances; *d, e:* cells stained along with several fasciculi of Meissner's plexus; *f, g:* ramified fibers; *j:* process of a cell that gives rise to a fascicle of fibers.

between three and eight processes. In addition bipolar cells have been observed, although they are the exception.

Regardless of the number of processes that these cells give rise to, they share a similar appearance. When stained completely, each process can be followed for quite some distance (figure 37, *a, b, c*). Furthermore, they ramify at variable distances from the cell body, giving rise to two, three, or even more varicose fibers (figure 37, *d, e*). The latter maintain a constant diameter as far as they can be traced, even after entering the fasciculi associated with the plexus. The largest processes frequently break up near their origin into a small bundle of fibers that are impossible to distinguish from those in the fasciculi of Meissner's plexus with which they intermingle (figure 37, *j*). In contrast, the thinnest fibers ramify very little, although I have been able to observe them branch two or three times as they cross the plexus at the level of a chiasma.

As far as the nature of these ganglion cell processes is concerned, let me simply note that, despite considerable effort, I have been unable to determine features that distinguish short dendritic processes from long processes or fibers of Remak.

b. Fibers of passage (figure 36, A and *c, e, f*)   In addition to cell processes, each ganglion contains a vast number of small and large fibers that enter by way of the fascicles.

Some of these fibers course through the ganglion to enter bundles leaving from the opposite side, while others pass from one fascicle to another, avoiding cellular regions. In addition, some fibers bifurcate upon entering the ganglion, and may thus supply branches to two different ganglia.

It is worth pointing out that quite often the cells and their processes do not contain silver chromate precipitates in individual preparations where fibers of passage are well stained, indicating that the latter have different characteristics.

c. Collaterals (figure 36, *c, e, f*)   Using apochromatic objectives, we have been able to distinguish exceedingly thin, highly varicose fibers within the ganglia. Such fibers wind among the cells, where they give rise to a rich, extremely complex plexus, rather than merely passing through the ganglia. Many of these fibers ramify along their course and end freely with swellings that contact cell bodies.

What is the origin of these unique fibers, which are such important structural elements of the ganglia? The pathways followed by some of them are so complex that I have been unable to determine their source. On the other hand, I am quite certain that some of them arise as collaterals from fibers passing through a ganglion. Two or even three such collaterals may arise at right or acute angles from such fibers, although it is worth emphasizing again that most fibers of passage lack collaterals.

The structure just described for Meissner's plexus (multipolar cells, fibers of passage, and collaterals) applies with only minor variations to Auerbach's plexus as well (figures 35, *a*, *g*; 37; and 39). I need mention just one fact that may be of significance. The only stained fibers in most preparations of Auerbach's plexus arise from the sympathetic system, and course through the mesenteric nerves to the ganglia and interganglionic fasciculi of the plexus (figure 38, B, A, C). It is even possible in some cases to follow one general sympathetic fiber through two or three ganglia in the plexus, thus establishing that most, if not all, of the fibers passing through the ganglia are simply extrinsic fibers of Remak that contact ganglion cells through collaterals and, perhaps, terminal arborizations as well. Such fibers may arise in the solar plexus or in abdominal sympathetic ganglia.

Are all of the fibers of passage derived from the sympathetic system? While this does not seem likely, definite proof is lacking.

Taken as a whole, my observations indicate that two elements contribute to the structure of intestinal ganglia: nerve cells with processes that distribute to smooth muscle fibers and to gland cells, and general sympathetic fibers that spread throughout the intestinal ganglia. The latter serve to place the sympathetic system, and perhaps other nerve centers as well, in contact with the intestinal plexuses.

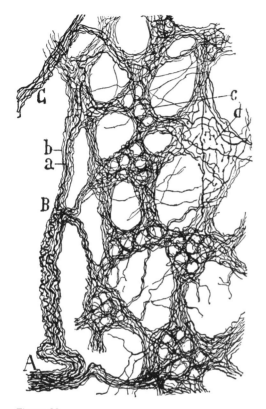

Figure 38
A section cut parallel to the muscular coat of the intestine in a newborn
mouse. Auerbach's plexus is seen in a frontal view along with ganglionic
thickenings, although the cells are not stained.
A: sympathetic nerve coursing along a branch of the mesenteric artery; B:
bifurcation of the sympathetic nerve; C: another afferent sympathetic nerve;
a: large sympathetic fibers; *b:* thin fibers; *c:* cavity for ganglion nerve cells; *d:*
collaterals ending within the ganglion.

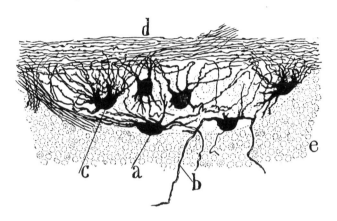

Figure 39
Longitudinal section through a ganglion of Auerbach's plexus from a four-day-old guinea pig.
a: deep cell with a small number of processes; *c:* cell with a vast number of processes; *b:* extraganglionic process of one cell; *d:* fibers of passage; *e:* transverse section through the circular layer of muscle fibers.

Interstitial Ganglia (figures 40 and 41)

These ganglia are represented by individual nerve cells that are scattered in large numbers between the acini of salivary glands (Fusari and Panarci), in the interstitial connective tissue of the pancreas (Cajal, Cl. Sala, and E. Müller), and finally, between the crypts of Lieberkühn and within the thickness of the intestinal villi (Drasch, Cajal, and Müller). I have also observed larger numbers of such cells along the inner face of the circular muscle fiber layer, where they form an extremely rich plexus (deep muscle plexus, figure 35, *b*) that extends to the contractile fibers by way of parallel fasciculi.

All of these cells are either fusiform, triangular, or stellate. Their processes are quite thick near their origin and begin immediately to divide and subdivide, forming a tangled plexus with the processes of neighboring visceral ganglia.

These processes appear to anastomose within a very dense plexus. It is in the intestine, therefore, that we first encounter

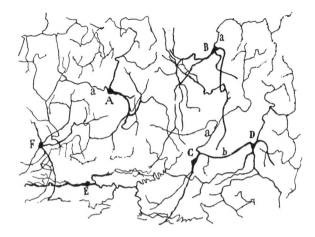

Figure 40
Interstitial nerve cells in the pancreas of the rabbit.
A: triangular cell giving rise to a thin, highly ramified process (*a*); B: a similar cell; C and D: cells that appear to anastomose by way of *b*; E: fusiform cell in the wall of an artery; F: stellate cell.

a true anastomotic plexus. However, it is important to bear in mind that these anastomoses are in all likelihood an illusion, and instead are nothing more than simple chiasmas or the intersection of fibers from neighboring fascicles.

The thinnest fibers appear to end freely by way of a varicosity either on smooth muscle fibers in the villi, mucosa, or circular layer, or on gland cells in the crypts of Lieberkühn or the glands of Brunner. These fibers end on the cytoplasm of the cells just mentioned. It is worth noting in passing that researchers using either methylene blue (Arnstein, Cajal, and Retzius) or silver chromate (Müller, Berkley, and Cajal) agree unanimously that sympathetic fibers end freely on both muscle and gland cells.

It is quite difficult, even in the best preparations, to determine whether fibers in the plexuses associated with villi and glands arise exclusively from interstitial cells or from Meissner's plexus. In summary, though my work on the visceral

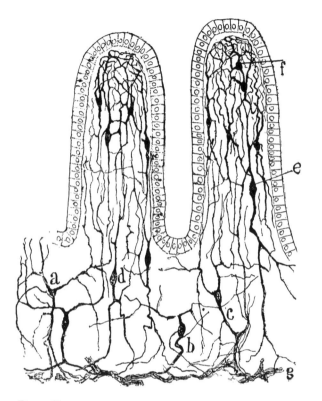

Figure 41
Nerve cells in the periglandular and villous plexuses of the guinea pig
intestine.
a, b, c: triangular or stellate cells of the glandular parenchyma; after coursing
for some distance, the relatively smooth processes break into actual fasciculi;
d: interglandular fusiform cell with ascending and descending processes; *e:*
fusiform cell deep within middle parts of a villus; *f:* triangular, stellate, or
occasionally spherical cell type in the distal part of a villus; *g:* Meissner's
plexus.

and interstitial ganglia is still far from complete, the following conclusions appear warranted.

1. Visceral ganglia contain multipolar cells whose processes course through plexuses to end on smooth muscle fibers or gland cells after ramifying many times.

2. Every ganglion also contains fibers of passage that probably arise in the sympathetic system, as well as collaterals that end among the nerve cells.

3. Every gland, and perhaps every group of smooth muscle fibers, no matter how small, contains interstitial nerve cells with processes that join the plexus formed by the visceral ganglia and sympathetic fibers.

4. In addition to forming an intersection for crossing fibers, every chiasma contains fibers of passage and the bifurcating processes of visceral ganglion cells.

5. There are no anastomoses between visceral ganglion cells or between fibers of passage or collaterals, and the same probably holds true for interstitial fibers as well.

Chapter 9
Neuroglia

Nerve centers harbor two kinds of supporting cells, *epithelial cells* and *neuroglial* or *spider cells*.

The ventricles associated with nerve centers are lined with a continuous sheet of *epithelial cells*. The nucleus of these elongated cells lies adjacent to the free surface of a ventricle, while one or more processes extend laterally from each cell into the neighboring gray or white matter, where they frequently diverge from one another and branch a number of times.

Epithelial cells throughout the length of the cerebrospinal axis are quite elongated during embryogenesis. In fact, they extend from the central cavity to the outer surface itself, just deep to the pia mater, where they form a cone-shaped ending with a peripheral base. Taken together, these cones form a kind of limiting membrane analogous to that formed by epithelial cells in the retina (Golgi). This arrangement is maintained through the entire lifespan in the brain of many vertebrates, including fish, reptiles, and amphibia, where the peripheral extensions of epithelial cells are the only neuroglial elements to be found. However, in the brains of birds and mammals, this epithelial layer atrophies in the sense that the divergent processes end in the middle of the gray or white matter rather than extending to the surface. The embryonic appearance of the epithelial neuroglia is preserved in just two regions: the olfactory mucosa and the retina.

The *spider cells* (which are properly referred to as neuroglial or Deiter's cells) are quite abundant in the white matter of nerve centers, within nerves (optic, olfactory, fiber layer of the retina, and so on), and in the ganglia of the sympathetic chain;

however they are much less frequent in the gray matter of the brain and spinal cord.

As Golgi demonstrated, neuroglial cells are small and give rise to a number of very thin, flexuous processes that ramify very little. These processes course in many directions and end freely, often on the surface of capillaries. The connective framework of nerve centers arises from the intermingled plexus of neuroglial processes, not an anastomotic plexus. The function of these processes may be related to the support and isolation of myelinated fibers; this appears to be a fundamental property in view of the fact that the processes are usually absent at the level of nerve cells themselves.

What is the origin of neuroglial cells? Based on the results of my own work, it would appear that neuroglial cells are nothing more than epithelial cells that have migrated from their usual position along the inner face of the various nerve centers, and are transformed into spider- or star-shaped cells by the atrophy of their central and peripheral processes and the formation of secondary processes. During this transformation, epithelial cells also divide and increase in number, as Lenhossék has recently shown.

Figure 42, which is taken from my own work on the spinal cord, illustrates the various phases of migration and transformation undergone by epithelial cells in the chick embryo. At one stage the displaced cells still maintain a peripheral radial process that ends near the pia mater, although this process subsequently atrophies; the same applies to the central process. The epithelial cell is then transformed into a neuroglial cell. Only epithelial cells associated with the ventral and dorsal medial grooves maintain their primitive shape and processes.

The complete transformation of epithelial cells into neuroglial elements takes place only in birds and mammals. The transition between the embryonic and adult spinal cord in birds and mammals is seen in amphibians (Lawdowski, Cl. Sala), fish (Retzius, Lenhossék, and others) and reptiles (Cajal) as the definitive, mature arrangement. Thus, in lower animals one observes epithelial cells in the process of migrating (figure

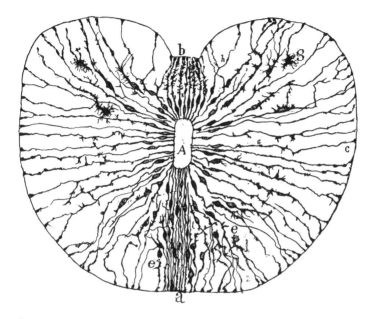

Figure 42
Epithelial cells and the origin of neuroglial cells as illustrated in the spinal cord of a nine-day chick embryo.

A: ependymal canal; *a:* epithelial cells of the dorsal median sulcus; *b:* epithelial cells of the ventral median fissure (these two groups of cells maintain their peripheral and central endings); *e:* displaced epithelial cells that have migrated to the dorsal horn; *f:* a displaced epithelial cell that has migrated to the ventral horn (the central processes of these two groups of cells have been completely lost, whereas the peripheral processes with conic endings near the pia mater are maintained); *g:* an epithelial cell that has almost become a neuroglial cell; a single process ending near the pia mater remains.

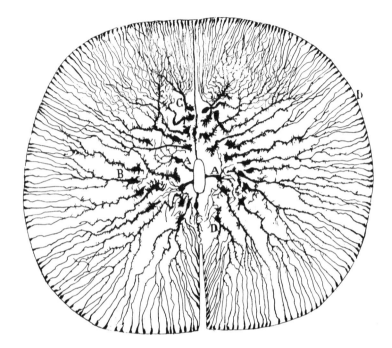

Figure 43
Neuroglial cells in the spinal cord of the adult frog (after Cl. Sala). All of the
cell bodies still lie within the periphery of the gray matter.
A: ependymal cells with their atrophied, ramified endings; B, C, D: neuroglial
cells at different stages of migration, and thus different distances from the
ependymal canal. Their central process is atrophied and considerably short-
ened, whereas their peripheral process is quite extended. The latter ramifies
and each branch ends in a conic bouton (I) just deep to the pia mater.

43) that nevertheless maintain a primitive morphology, as well as a peripheral, radial process that ends near the pia mater. Cells whose perikaryon and nucleus remain to line the ependymal cavity display an atrophied peripheral process with ramifications that generally remain within the gray matter. Thus, while the central process of neuroglial cells in reptiles and amphibians atrophies and contracts, the peripheral process atrophies and contracts in cells that maintain their original position (ependymal cells).

The adult spinal cord of amphibians (Lawdowski and C. Sala) and reptiles (Cajal) constitutes a transition stage between the embryonic and adult spinal cord in mammals because here epithelial cells in the process of migration maintain a primitive morphology and display a peripheral radial process that ends near the pia mater. This transitory stage has also been examined in the human spinal cord by Lenhossék.

In an earlier study I raised the possibility that certain neuroglial cells may be intimately associated with blood vessels arising from either an endothelial proliferation or a migration of connective tissue cells into regions of the nervous system. However, I have observed the same phenomenon, namely the existence of a few thin, divergent processes that arise from the endothelium of capillaries in neural centers, in other tissues such as the tongue, dermal mucosa, and muscle. This leads me to believe that there is a single mechanism involved in the histogenesis of neuroglial cells: the migration and differentiation of typical epithelial cells. The significance of the above-mentioned perivascular expansions, which have also been confirmed by Lachi in the spinal cord of the embryonic chick, is still not clear to me.

Chapter 10

Development of Nerve Cells

The work in which His successfully followed the various phases that ectodermal cells go through in their transformation to nerve cells of the mammalian embryo illuminated the interesting problem of how this important cell type develops. We shall now summarize what is known about this topic, based on the most recent information.

The epithelium of the ectodermal medullary groove (the medullary plate) contains two types of elements: elongated epithelial cells, which stretch from one surface of the membrane to the other, and spherical cells, which lie near the outer face in a groove that is formed in the membrane itself. The latter are referred to as *germinal cells* and arise through the active karyokinesis of elements that later form neuroblasts or undifferentiated nerve cells. The epithelium is also the only source of cells that later form the ependyma and neuroglia.

Germinal Cells, Neuroblasts, and Development of the Axon
When the medullary groove closes to form a tube, the walls of the embryonic spinal cord become thicker and undergo an important phase of differentiation.

A large number of germinal cells migrate toward the outer half of the medullary wall. Along the way they are transformed into *neuroblasts*, that is, into piriform cells with an oval cell body that is directed either dorsally or medially, and a simple, relatively thick process that grows continuously and crosses the thickness of the primitive gray matter; this process is the primordial axon.

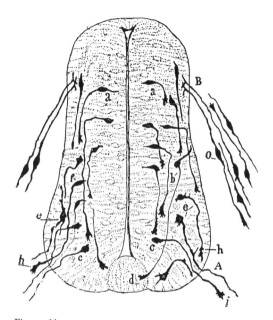

Figure 44
A section through the spinal cord of a chick embryo on the third day of incubation.

A: ventral root; B: dorsal root; *a:* very young neuroblasts; *b:* more developed (probably commissural) neuroblasts; *c:* neuroblasts that contribute an axon to the ventral roots; *d:* growth cone of a commissural axon; *h, i:* growth cones of fibers in the ventral roots; *e:* ventral root cells that already display rudimentary dendrites; *o:* ganglion cells.

It is not possible to observe the growing tip of an axon in preparations stained with carmine or hematoxylin. Because of this, His was unable to distinguish clearly such endings and could not refute Hensen, who denied that nerve fibers grow toward the periphery because no one had yet observed the tip of an axon in the process of growing.

My observations in the chick embryo (on the third day of incubation) have led to a definitive resolution of this problem, and favor the theory proposed by His rather than that put forward by Hensen. I have demonstrated that as every primordial axon stretches across the spinal cord, it ends in a special conical swelling, the *growth cone*, with a base that faces the periphery and is garnished with a large number of thin protrusions and lamellar processes that might be considered a form of rudimentary terminal arborization. The growth cone is like an amoebic mass that acts as a battering ram to spread the elements along its path, insinuating its lamellar processes between them. Figure 45 shows neuroblasts as they appear in the chick spinal cord on the third and fourth days of incubation. Here we can also observe a group of cells in the ventral horn that send their growth cones to the ventral root, as well as another group of neuroblasts scattered throughout most of the gray matter whose growth cones are directed toward the ventral commissure. Finally, a small number of neuroblasts insert their processes into peripheral regions of the spinal cord that will later form territories occupied by myelinated bundles. These processes either bend or undergo a T-shaped division and then invariably assume a longitudinal course.

As we shall see, the epithelium does not remain inactive while the germinal cells undergo these metamorphoses.

Epithelial Cells and Connective or Neuroglial Formations
Each epithelial cell should in fact be thought of as consisting of two parts, one outer and one inner. The latter has a relatively smooth contour and harbors the nucleus. It is separated from the processes of neighboring epithelial cells by elongated spaces that come to be populated by large numbers of neu-

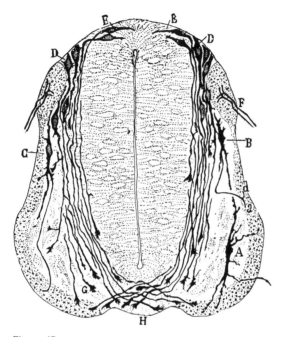

Figure 45
A section through the upper spinal cord of a chick embryo on the fourth day
of incubation.
A: ventral root cell; B: ventrolateral funicular cell; C: ventral funicular cell; D:
piriform neuroblasts with an axon that ends in a growth cone at the level of
the ventral commissure; E: young nerve cells that are still shaped like spongioblasts; F: dorsal root; G: growth cone; H: embryonic ventral commissure.

roblasts (the columnar layer of His). The inner part is garnished with many short collateral processes analogous to spines. These processes make contact with those from neighboring epithelial cells, thus forming a spongy framework with interstices that will serve as passages for nerve fibers in the white matter (the marginal velum or *Randschleier* of His). According to His, these interstices lie ventral to the developing nerve fibers and thus play an extremely important role as a kind of preexisting set of channels that the ends of the axons are forced to pass through. However, it would appear to me that the epithelial cell processes, and thus the interstitial spaces of His' marginal velum, lie dorsal rather than ventral to the developing fiber bundles. In addition, I have observed that during all of the important stages of neural differentiation in the brain and retina the growth and distribution of axons take place at a time when the epithelial cells are still simple radial fibers without lateral processes.

Be that as it may, His' theory that the growth of nerve fibers always takes place in the direction of least resistance, and that this direction is determined by preexisting connective or neuroglial structures, is an ingenious hypothesis worthy of further examination.

It may, however, be preferable to consider that a kind of positive *chemotaxis* acts on neuroblasts and is exerted by trophic factors elaborated by other neural, epithelial, or muscular elements.[1]

The force that drives a neuroblast to send its axon toward a muscle, for example, can also be explained by the existence of different electrical states in the neuroblast and muscle, an hypothesis recently advanced by Strasser. The influence of a negative electrical state in a muscle fiber or any other cell type that receives the terminal arborization of an axon may produce a positive electrical state in the outer pole of the neuroblast

1. For further details, see Ramon y Cajal's study on the "Retina of Vertebrates" that appeared in *La Cellule*, 1892.

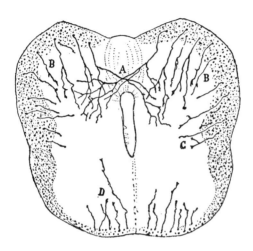

Figure 46
A section through the embryonic spinal cord.
A: germinal cells; B: inner part of the epithelial cells (pillar layer); C: outer part of the epithelial cells (reticular layer or marginal velum); *n:* neuroblast (of His).

that would induce it to move in the direction of greatest potential difference.

Development of Dendrites and Collaterals
The final stages of neuroblast development have been examined with the rapid Golgi method. The independent observations of Lenhossék and myself on the chick spinal cord completed the cycle of work begun by His in demonstrating how and when dendritic arborizations and axon collaterals arise.

As soon as the axon forms, a short polar expansion that may possibly be regarded as the outline of a dendrite can be seen. However, this polar expansion is often missing, and dendrites are normally first recognized as large, spiny outgrowths from any part of the neuroblast cell body, or from the region that gives rise to the axon itself. The free end often bears a varicosity.

In turn, axon collaterals arise several days after the formation of dendrites. They begin as a short process that emerges at a right angle and has a varicosity on the end.

The first collaterals to appear in the chick spinal cord (on the fourth to fifth days of incubation) are found in the ventral funiculus; during the following days, collaterals can be seen to sprout in the dorsal columns and lateral funiculus.

I have already pointed out that axon bifurcations (T- or Y-shaped fibers) begin to form well before this time, during the growth phase of the primitive nerve fibers.

It is quite easy to focus on the *growth of nerve fibers in the ventral roots toward the muscles* in preparations of the vertebral column from chicks during the fifth to seventeenth days of incubation. In general, the roots are completely formed by the fifth day, when the fibers have developed to such an extent that it is impossible to find their endings within the thickness of the roots themselves. In fact, they are already bound to neighboring muscle masses by way of varicosities. An extraordinary number of ramifications arise along the course of each axon. For example, I have observed a large motor fiber supply more than thirty terminal branches, each directed to a single muscle fiber, in a seventeen-day-old chick embryo. The motor end plates that had not yet formed were represented by a varicose fiber that ended in a small sphere applied to the muscle cell. In some instances the nerve fiber had begun to produce a number of short processes, the initial parts of the end plate terminal arborization.

The above description applies to most nerve cells. There are, however, some that behave differently and show certain developmental peculiarities that deserve brief description.

Spinal Ganglion Cells
As is well known, these cells are unipolar in mammals, birds, amphibians, and reptiles. It is only in fish that they display a

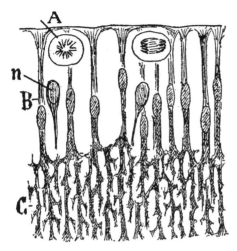

Figure 47
The spinal cord of a chick embryo sectioned on the seventh day of incubation.
A: collaterals in the ventral funiculus that traverse the ventral commissure; B:
less developed collaterals that end in a growth cone; C: the most embryonic
collaterals in the lateral funiculus; D: collaterals in the dorsal funiculus.

bipolar shape, like olfactory cells in the nasal fossa or spiral
ganglion cells in the cochlea.

It might appear that there is an essential difference in the
morphology of sensory ganglion cells when comparing the
higher vertebrates with fish. However, His discovered a very
interesting fact: sensory ganglion cells are bipolar in the mammalian embryo just as in adult fish. This greatly reduces the
difference that appears to separate them.

There are two primordial extensions from these cells. The
inner process is generally thinner and grows along the dorsal
root to enter the dorsal funiculus of the spinal cord, where I
have established that it bifurcates into ascending and descending branches. I also discovered a growth cone that is directed
toward the spinal cord on this branch of the cells in the three-
day chick embryo. The outer branch grows toward the periph-

ery and mingles with motor fibers before ending in the skin, mucosae, or Golgi tendon organs.

Bipolar cells undergo modifications that are proportional to the increasing volume of the spinal ganglion. According to His, and confirmed in avian and reptilian embryos by me as well as by Lenhossék, C. Sala, Retzius, E. Müller, and van Gehuchten, the regions of cytoplasm that give rise to the two processes move closer together, gradually fuse, and then on one side of the cell form a pedicle of cytoplasm that constitutes the only support for the two nerve fibers. The entire transition from the bipolar phase to the unipolar phase is clearly illustrated in figure 48, which is taken from a spinal ganglion in the fourteen-day chick embryo. An examination of this figure gives the impression that there is a tendency for cells to migrate toward the periphery of the ganglion, with the center reserved for nerve fibers and bifurcation pedicles.

These facts prove that there are transitory developmental phases in vertebrate cellular ontogenesis and that the early phase is a permanent feature of adult fish.

Furthermore, Lenhossék has also shown that the unipolar cells lie side by side with bipolar cells in certain fish (*Pristurus* embryos). Thus, it is clear that the transition from bipolar to unipolar has already begun in certain fish. Taken as a whole, the results of this work indicate that every sensory cell is or was bipolar in the embryo. Therefore, every sensory cell always has two processes: a peripheral process that gathers centripetal stimuli near the surface of the body, and a central fiber, which is usually thinner, that is involved in conducting the stimulus gathered by the peripheral process to a nerve center.

When viewed in this way, sensory cells form a well-defined cell type that readily includes (1) spinal ganglion cells, (2) bipolar cells of the olfactory mucosa, and (3) bipolar cells in the retina and the organ of hearing.

The fusiform cells discovered recently by Lenhossék in the skin of the earthworm, which have been confirmed by Retzius, also fall into this category. These cells have a large peripheral

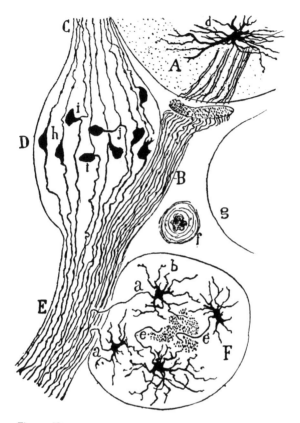

Figure 48
Spinal and sympathetic ganglia in the cervical region of a chick embryo on the seventeenth day of incubation.
A: spinal cord with a ventral root cell, *d;* B: ventral or motor root; C: dorsal or sensory root; D: spinal ganglion; E: cervical spinal nerve; F: sympathetic ganglion; *a:* sympathetic axons forming the rami communicantes and coursing toward the corresponding spinal nerve; *b:* dendrite of a sympathetic cell; *e:* sympathetic axons coursing vertically to enter the longitudinal commissure of the ganglion; *h:* fusiform cell in the spinal ganglion; *i:* transition from a bipolar to a unipolar cell in the spinal ganglion; *f:* definitive unipolar cell; *g:* cross section of an artery.

process that ends on the surface of the epidermis, and a thin central process that courses through the body of the animal to the ganglionic chain where it bifurcates into ascending and descending branches, like fibers in the vertebrate dorsal roots. Thus, these unique cells correspond to vertebrate spinal ganglion cells, with the only difference being that in worms the cell bodies, which are derived from the ectodermal layer, have not yet been pulled into the center of the body to form ganglia.

Cells with a Dendritic Tuft
Cerebellar Purkinje cells, cortical pyramidal cells, and retinal ganglion cells all pass through the neuroblast phase. However, their dendrites are formed in a specific way that is important to understand. The first process to appear after the axon is usually the peripheral tuft, which is quite irregular and varicose. This peripheral dendritic bouquet later distances itself from the cell body, and the principal dendritic trunk is thus formed. The last stage of development includes the formation of collateral branches from the trunk and basal processes from the cell body.

These basal processes persist and undergo further elaboration in cortical pyramidal cells. The same is not true, however, for the Purkinje cells and retinal ganglion cells; they appear at about the same time as the principal trunk and then atrophy and disappear completely.

Granule Cells of the Cerebellum
These cells undergo an extremely curious metamorphosis that is somewhat reminiscent of unipolar spinal ganglion cells.

As is well known, there is a special zone above the molecular layer in the cerebellum of newborn mammals (mouse, rabbit, dog, human, and so on) that contains a dense complement of small cells called superficial granule cells. In addition, the number of such cells decreases steadily as the cerebellum develops, and at a certain time during the adult period they disappear completely.

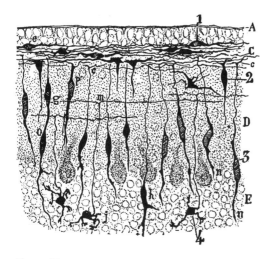

Figure 49
A section through the cerebellum of a twelve-day-old mouse. The development of granule cells is illustrated.
A: superficial layer of granule cells; C: layer of horizontal bipolar cells; D: molecular layer; E: layer of true or deep granule cells; 1: first stage of granule cell development (horizontal bipolar cell); 2: second stage of granule cell development (vertical bipolar cell that gives rise to a descending process from the perikaryon); 3: third stage of granule cell development (the ascending axon is quite obvious and the deep part of the cell body has arrived in the deep granular layer); 4: fourth stage of granule cell development (mature granule cell).

What population of cells decreases in direct proportion to the increase in true granule cells deep in the cerebellum?

When I began studying the cerebellum, I noted that deeper parts of the superficial granular layer consist of horizontally oriented, fusiform bipolar cells with long processes that resemble axons that are all arranged parallel to the longitudinal axis of the folium. This would have led one to believe that parallel fibers analogous to those arising from the axon of deep granule cells are involved. In fact, these bipolar cells are nothing more than primitive forms of the deep granule cells! Due to their migration through the subjacent molecular layer, which is opposite to the migration of bipolar spinal ganglion cells that proceeds from a central to a peripheral location, these cells reach the depths of the cerebellar folia where they assume all of the characteristics of adult granule cells. Before arriving in the depths of a folium, these cells pass through the following stages. (1) A dendritic process descends from the body of a horizontal bipolar cell, and gradually carries the cell body (with the nucleus) along with it toward the depths of the cerebellum. (2) This process, which advances perpendicularly through the thickness of the molecular layer, has an elongated appearance and gives rise to two expansions. One ascends to the superficial part of the molecular layer where it forms a parallel fiber, while the other descends to end freely near the deep granular zone. (3) When the cell, which can be thought of as being delivered by and through the descending process, arrives in the deep granular layer the ascending process becomes thinner and assumes the appearance of an axon that ends as a parallel fiber. The cell body then gives rise to three or more short processes that soon become the dendrites that are so characteristic of deep granule cells. This developmental history reveals two interesting facts. First, we can see that the parallel fiber becomes, in a way, permanently established in the region occupied originally by the two processes of a horizontal bipolar cell, just as I observed in the case of spinal ganglion cells. And second, the ascending axon and the fingerlike processes of the granule cell arise through a mechanism that involves proto-plasmic stretching.

Retinal Amacrine Cells
Nerve cells that lack an axon do not pass through the neuro-blast stage, as is the case for nonneuronal amacrine cells in the retina, which lack an axon. Here, a large bouquet of short, varicose fibers is first elaborated on the inner face of the cell body. This is merely an outline of the terminal arborization. Later, the cell body becomes elongated in the longitudinal plane, and the terminal arborization is suspended from a trunk that arises on the inner surface of the cell body. This, in any event, is the developmental history of certain amacrine cells in the retina of chickens and rabbits.

The nonneuronal amacrine cells of the retina are not the only elements in the animal kingdom with these morpholog-ical and developmental features. At least on the basis of shape, they are in fact rather common, and may be regarded as the morphologically defined developmental stage achieved by in-vertebrate nerve cells. Thus, according to the work of Bieder-mann, Retzius, and Lenhossék, nerve cells in the ganglia of invertebrates (crustaceans and worms) are most commonly unipolar. Their single process is generally quite thick and gives rise to collaterals that end freely within the ganglia. When the cell is multipolar, all of the processes appear to display the same features, that is, they all appear to be axonal (Retzius). In contrast, the cells in vertebrate nerve centers undergo im-portant transformations that carry them far from the primitive shape of neuroblasts so common in the nerve centers of in-vertebrates. Nevertheless, some primitive forms that more or less resemble neuroblasts with no differentiation of their pro-cesses still persist in the adult vertebrate. These include the amacrine cells of the retina, as we have just seen, as well as granule cells in the olfactory bulb, visceral and intestinal sym-pathetic cells (Auerbach's, Meissner's, and other plexuses), and probably certain cells in the first layer of the cerebral cortex.

Chapter 11
General Conclusions

The following considerations emerge from the facts outlined in the foregoing synthesis.

1. The most general conclusion related to the cellular morphology of nerve centers is the absence of continuity between neural, epithelial, and neuroglial processes. The neural elements are true cellular entities or neurons, to use Waldeyer's term.

2. Because there is no actual continuity, currents must be transmitted from one cell to another by way of contiguity or contact, as in the splicing of two telegraph wires. This contact takes place between the terminal arborizations and collaterals of axons on one side, and the cell bodies and dendritic arborizations on the other. When no dendrites are present, as in the case of retinal amacrine cells, unipolar spinal ganglion cells, and invertebrate unipolar cells, axonal arborizations are applied only to the surface of the cell body.

3. The probable direction of current flow in neurons with both types of processes is *cellulipetal* in the dendrites and *cellulifugal* in the axon. Cellulifugal flow appears to take place in the process or processes of cells with a single type of expansion (amacrine cells, and so on). In these cells the receptive or cellulipetal surface is represented by the thin crust of cytoplasm surrounding the nucleus.

4. The peripheral process of bipolar cells is large and should be regarded as dendritic because it functions to gather currents (cellulipetal flow). Examples of such cells include sensory bipolar cells in worms (according to Lenhossék and Retzius);

auditory, olfactory, and retinal cells; and sensory bipolar cells in the spinal ganglia of fish.

In the unipolar spinal ganglion cells of amphibians, reptiles, birds, and mammals, the peripheral branch of the single process arising from the cell body could be viewed as a dendrite or organ of cellulipetal transmission, whereas the thinner central process is like a nerve fiber or organ of cellulifugal transmission. The trunk that contains the two processes before they bifurcate is not present early in embryogenesis (His); it forms later as the result of cell body migration. Therefore, on morphological and developmental grounds, it constitutes part of the cell body rather than a nerve fiber.

5. Golgi and his students would have us believe that dendrites simply play a role in nutrition, acting as a system of rootlets for sucking up the plasma exuded from capillaries. However, in my opinion, they function as conductors just like axons. Golgi put forward two facts in support of his thesis: a tendency for dendrites to cluster around blood vessels, and connections between dendrites and neuroglial cells. However, these observations have not been confirmed by me or by van Gehuchten, Koelliker, Lenhossék, Retzius, Schaefer, and others.

First, the olfactory glomeruli of lower vertebrates have neither blood vessels nor glial cells. In spite of this, the dendrites of mitral cells and other cell types end in these glomeruli, as in mammals.

Second, the inner plexiform layer of the retina, which contains the ganglion cell dendrites, lacks both capillaries and neuroglial cells in lower vertebrates. Nevertheless, the well-known arrangement of these dendrites, as well as their connections with bipolar cells, are not altered in the slightest degree.

And third, every region of the gray matter that contains nerve terminals also contains dendritic arborizations. In addition, the reverse is true: no region that contains dendrites does not contain the terminal arborizations of axons as well. Koelliker and several others have expressed some doubt about the latter point, citing the existence of dendrites in regions of the brain and spinal cord that consist of white matter, which contains only myelinated fibers of passage and thus provides no substrate for communication between cells. This objection has lost its force in light of the following results of my work. (1) special collaterals end in the white matter of both the brain and spinal cord; (2) these regions contain, or may contain, unmyelinated nerve fibers that give rise to characteristic terminal branches; (3) regions that have been said to contain only dendrites (such as certain planes in the granular layer of the optic lobe of reptiles, amphibians, and fish) also harbor a large number of terminal arborizations arising from unmyelinated axons.

My recent observations on the spinal cord of reptiles and amphibians also merit attention from this point of view. The dendrites of cells in the ventral horn are enormously long in these animals. After forming bundles that radiate through the white matter, they form an exceedingly thick perimedullary plexus around the white matter, just below the pia mater. I first reported this plexus in reptiles, and it was subsequently observed in amphibians by Lawdowski. Quite recently, C. Sala has studied these plexuses quite carefully in amphibian larvae. In summary, this plexus contains the endings of certain peripheral collaterals that arise from myelinated fibers in the white matter, as well as the terminals of certain unmyelinated fibers. I have also recently observed the presence in the outermost zone of the lateral funiculus of true fusiform nerve cells, which have a rostrocaudal orientation and branched dendrites that are contacted by the peripheral collaterals mentioned above. These observations were made in the cervical spinal cord of sixteen-day-old chick embryos.

6. The extreme length of certain dendritic trunks (such as those arising from cortical pyramidal cells and Purkinje cells), combined with a wealth of lateral and basal dendrites, appears to be necessary for gathering currents from a correspondingly large number of axonal arborizations. It would appear that the fine projections and interspinal notches found on many dendritic arborizations represent contact sites for axon terminals.

Chapter 12
The Golgi Method

Golgi envisioned the use of two methods for studying nerve centers: one has been called the black-staining or silver chromate method, and the other the gray-staining or mercuric chloride method.

In principle, the black-staining method, which is now the most common approach used by neurologists, consists of hardening pieces of neural tissue in potassium bichromate or Müller's fluid and then exposing them to the action of silver nitrate. The latter reagent produces a reddish-black silver chromate precipitate in a small number of cells.

In the gray-staining method based on the use of mercury salts, pieces of neural tissue are treated and hardened with mercuric chloride in Müller's fluid. A metallic precipitate, which appears gray or black under transmitted light, forms within certain fibers and cells and allows them to be seen quite clearly because they are highlighted distinctly against a translucent yellow background.

As just mentioned, the silver chromate method is the more widely used of the two, and the most important discoveries have been made with it. In general, the mercuric chloride method has been used as a control for the results obtained with the alternative method.

Let us first examine the silver chromate method, which includes two variants that I shall refer to as the rapid and slow procedures.

Golgi preferred the slow procedure for his studies on the brain and cerebellum. In this case, hardening takes place in Müller's fluid and potassium dichromate without osmic acid.

The pieces of tissue are stored in hardening fluids for one to two months before they are exposed to silver nitrate.

A number of other workers, including myself, Koelliker, von Lenhossék, van Gehuchten, Tartuferi, and Retzius have preferred to use the rapid procedure, where the hardening fluid consists of a mixture of potassium dichromate and osmic acid solutions. This mixture allows for a considerable shortening of the hardening time to two to six days, and also produces staining that is even more delicate than the slow procedure.

Rapid Silver Chromate Procedure

The rapid silver chromate method will now be described in detail, along with small variations that I and others have introduced to the original procedure used by Golgi.

1. To begin, use scissors or a razor to cut neural tissue into pieces that are no more than 4 mm thick. Then immerse the pieces for 24, 48, or 56 hours in the following solution:

Potassium dichromate	3 g
Distilled water	100 cc
1% osmic acid	30 to 35 cc

The volume of hardening fluid should be proportional to the number of pieces in it. Thus, three 4 mm thick pieces require about 30 cc, that is, about 10 cc of the osmium-dichlorate solution for each 4 mm piece.

It matters little whether the pieces are exposed to light or kept in the dark during the hardening process. On the other hand, temperature does play an important role. In my experience temperatures between 20° and 25°C are the most favorable. However, good results can be obtained at 8° to 9°C, although the pieces must remain in the solution longer.

2. The pieces are removed from the above solution, washed rapidly in distilled water, and plunged into a large volume of silver nitrate solution (0.50 or 0.75 g per 100 cc). They remain in the silver solution for 24 hours to several days, although I usually remove them after 36 hours.

When dealing with brain or spinal cord tissue that is more or less fully developed, I add one or two drops of formic acid to each 300 cc of silver nitrate solution. It is my impression that this renders the preparations more translucent and leads to more extensive impregnation. I have not found it useful to add formic acid to tissues that are difficult to stain, such as organs at an early stage of development. In fact, I almost never use formic acid.

There appears to be no influence of light and temperature on pieces of tissue in the silver bath, and I routinely stain under normal conditions of lighting and temperature. However, it is wise to keep tissue in the dark if it is to be processed several days after immersion in the silver solution. If this is not done, irregular shrinkage occurs in the piece of tissue, as pointed out by van Gehuchten.

3. Sections of the tissue block should be rather thick so that stained elements can be followed as far as possible. To make sections, the tissue block should be coated with celloidin or paraffin and then mounted either between two pieces of stripped elder bark or in a piece of cork. The resulting assemblage is then placed on a microtome, such as those developed by Ranvier, Reichert, Schanze, and Becker.

I proceed as follows. First, I dehydrate the surface of the tissue block by immersing it in 95 percent alcohol (40 percent Cartier) for one to two minutes, then dry it with blotting paper, and finally place it on a flat piece of hard paraffin. Then, with the point of a scalpel or needle heated in a flame, I quickly melt the paraffin around the inner part of the tissue block to embed and firmly attach it to the paraffin. It is essential to perform this little maneuver quickly to avoid drying of the tissue block. The part of the neural tissue that remains exposed is quickly dipped in 95 percent alcohol, and the whole block is taken to the microtome. Sections are then cut, taking care to wet the knife with 95 percent alcohol (40 percent Cartier).

4. The sections are collected in 95 percent alcohol, and taken through five or six changes over a period of not more than an

hour. After longer times, the alcohol causes a bleaching of the thinnest fibers.

5. The sections are removed from the alcohol and placed in a bath of oil of cloves for half an hour or less. They should be mounted as soon as they have cleared and become transparent.

6. The sections are placed on glass slides and the excess oil of cloves is removed with blotting paper applied with moderate pressure. Then, small amounts of xylol are poured over the sections to remove the last of the oil.

7. The xylol is drained by simply placing the slides vertically, and the sections are then covered with a relatively thin solution of Dammar resin in xylol and oriented in parallel rows with a needle. The sections are dried with the slides positioned horizontally, protected from dust. After an hour or two, when the first layer of Dammar is almost dry, the sections are covered with a second layer, and this procedure is repeated until the surface of the sections is covered entirely with a smooth layer of the resin.

Cover glasses should be avoided because their use produces very rapid alterations. According to Sanassa, this is due to diffusion currents that remove deposits of silver chromate from impregnated elements.

It is also necessary to leave the preparations uncovered, although this is inconvenient and requires certain precautions to protect them. Once the Dammar resin is dry, the preparations should be protected from light and dust.

Unfortunately, the sections cannot be maintained in their original state, in spite of these precautions. After two or three years the background of the sections becomes deeply colored and the silver chromate diffuses to a greater or lesser extent around stained elements. However, the preparations should not be considered lost. Their beauty and clarity are diminished, but brighter illumination overcomes the inconvenient increase in background coloration. In general, the thicker the section, the easier it is for darkening and ruin to strike. I have been able to save sections of average thickness for over four years with no signs of alteration.

A variety of procedures have been devised for rendering Golgi preparations indelible. Treating the sections with hydrobromic acid (Greppin) or gold chloride (Obrégia) does preserve the cell bodies and dendrites, although thin nerve fibers fade to some extent, and may even disappear completely.

In summary, the conditions necessary for good preservation of the sections are as follows: the sections should not be too thick; they should be washed thoroughly in alcohol to remove all traces of silver nitrate; they must remain desiccated under a relatively thin layer of Dammar resin; they cannot be cover slipped; and they must be stored in darkness.

Double Impregnation Procedure

1. The tissue blocks are removed from the silver bath and dried with blotting paper. They are then placed in an osmium-dichromate solution like that used above, although it may contain more dichromate. The solution contains:

Potassium dichromate	6 to 7 g
Distilled water	100 cc
Osmic acid	30 to 35 cc

Tissue remains in this solution for one to two days. If one is concerned that the tissue may harden excessively and become too fragile, the amount of osmic acid can be reduced.

2. The pieces of tissue are removed from this solution, dried with blotting paper, and soaked for 24 hours in a 0.5 or 0.75 percent silver nitrate solution, just as with the first impregnation.

In a successful preparation the cells and nerve fibers are stained very clearly against a pale yellow background. The cells and thicker dendrites are stained black, while the axons are brown or reddish brown, and the thinnest collaterals are yellowish red. Neuroglial cells are usually dark red, although they may also appear completely black.

Silver chromate is not deposited on the surface of cells, as Sehrwald and Rossbach suggested, but is instead found diffusely throughout the thickness of the cytoplasm.

The precious advantage of this method is that only a small number of cells are stained, and these are usually separated by unstained elements. This fortunate quirk lends the neatness and clarity of a diagram to a good preparation. In addition, the transparent background allows very thick sections to be examined. This is another considerable advantage because it allows the longest nerve cell processes to be followed in one and the same section.

In cells with a small amount of cytoplasm, the nucleus is visible, its coffee color apparent against a black background.

Rules Concerning the Use of the Rapid Silver Chromate Method
The following rules complement the technical information just provided. They can serve as a guide to anyone wishing to use the Golgi method, and, if observed, can eliminate many trials and tribulations.

1. The rapid Golgi method only yields consistent, totally reproducible results in nerve centers during a period around the time that myelination takes place. If the age of the animal is such that the myelination phase of a particular nerve center is greatly preceded, or almost all of the myelin sheaths have already formed, staining of the cells and fibers will be very inconsistent.

2. It should not be assumed that all nerve centers stain equally with the rapid Golgi procedure.

Based on a large number of experiments, I have classified the various parts of the nervous system with regard to their staining consistency. Ammon's horn and the cerebral cortex of the eight-day-old rabbit, and the spinal cord of the seven-to-fourteen-day-old chick embryo stain most consistently and completely. I would invite anyone interested in becoming familiar with the Golgi method to start with an examination of the regions just mentioned. Other more difficult regions can then be studied much more easily. I should also add that excellent preparations of these regions can be assured if two conditions are met: the appropriate volume of hardening solution, and time of hardening. The olfactory bulb of rabbits, dogs, and other young animals, and the cerebellum of young animals (for example, the eight-day-old guinea pig, and the month-old rabbit and rat) fall in a second class. Here, the reaction is complete but not as consistent as in the regions mentioned above. Finally, the sympathetic ganglia, retina, olfactory mucosa, sensory and motor endings, auditory nerve endings, and so on must be regarded as difficult to stain.

3. It is important to choose the most appropriate animal to obtain good results. The size of the region to be studied, its relationship to other centers, and perhaps certain unknown chemical features may all favor or interfere with the reaction, and may increase or decrease the formation of irregular deposits. For example, the retina is better stained in birds and large reptiles than in amphibians, fish, and mammals; and the cortex of an eight-day-old rabbit is stained much better than that of the rat, guinea pig, albino mouse, dog, and so on at a comparable developmental stage. Furthermore, the spinal cord of avian embryos reacts to silver chromate more completely and consistently than does the spinal cord of reptilian and mammalian embryos, the optic lobe in birds stains better than the superior colliculi in mammals, and so on.

4. The earlier the developmental stage of the region to be studied, the less time it needs to spend in the hardening solution. For example, a good reaction can be obtained in the chick spinal cord from the fifth to sixth days of incubation after 24 hours of hardening, whereas three days in the osmium-dichromate solution is necessary for satisfactory staining from the fourteenth to fifteenth days of incubation. Similarly, the cerebellum of a newborn rabbit needs only 24 hours of hardening, while that of a one-month-old rabbit yields well-stained sections only after two to three days of hardening.

5. It is useful whenever possible to include a small region of tissue around the organ or part of an organ that is to be

hardened. This avoids irregular deposits on the surface of the region of interest. For example, the entire vertebral column is left around the chick spinal cord if the column is thin, as it is during the first days of incubation. On the other hand, only a part of the vertebral column is included if it is too large.

It is always necessary to leave the pia mater on the brain. And, as Sehrwald suggests, it is sometimes advantageous to coat the surface of a tissue block with a layer of gelatin before submersion in the silver solution.

6. One knows that the hardening is incomplete if the sections display a uniform red background with incompletely stained cells and fibers. On the other hand, the hardening has been extended too long when the background is light yellow and no elements, or only a few nerve fibers, stand out in black.

7. One can also recognize that the block was too lightly hardened if there is a virtual absence of stained cells, and an almost exclusive staining of nerve fibers. This accident may be corrected by returning to a second impregnation. The same would apply to double and even triple staining of organs that are difficult to impregnate, such as the retina, sympathetic ganglia, intestinal ganglia, auditory endings, and so on. One rarely obtains virtually complete staining with a single impregnation.

8. It is necessary to optimize a number of staining conditions to obtain reliable results, particularly when attempting to clarify new problems. It is also necessary to proceed by carrying out one trial after another. The organ of interest is divided into several pieces and a different hardening time is applied to each. This is an essential part of the silver chromate method. For example, one of the pieces is left in the osmium dichromate solution for 24 hours, a second for 36 hours, a third for 48 hours, another for three days, another for four days, and so on. Finally, all of the hardened pieces undergo double or even triple impregnation. One may in this way determine quickly the optimal conditions for successful impregnation of an organ. *Nevertheless, it must be pointed out that*

the experience and competency of the investigator in determining these conditions are essential; the beginner can only hope to achieve success with difficult impregnations after many long months of repeated trials and perseverance.

The gold chloride method is similar to the Golgi method, and is difficult if not impossible in the hands of a beginner. On the other hand, it proved a docile instrument in the hands of Ranvier, Golgi, Loewit, Retzius, Rollett, and others, who made important discoveries with it.

9. The following two conditions should play a major role in the way studies are carried out.

Silver chloride has the peculiar feature of staining only a very small number of fibers and cells at a time, and it is not uncommon to find that cells that have resisted impregnation despite months of persevering efforts suddenly appear marvelously stained. It is also important to point out that in any study based on the Golgi method, preparations must be repeated over and over. First, this allows one to establish the complete structure of an organ from the partial information in each preparation. And second, the repeated observation of a particular histological feature in a number of different preparations is the absolute guarantee of its reality. One thus avoids describing arrangements due to chance or a caprice of incomplete staining, arrangements that inexperienced observers all too often regard as definitive, constant features of an organ's structure.

10. Every Golgi preparation of a nerve center should always be compared with preparations of the same adult tissue stained with the Weigert-Pal method, as well as with carmine and aniline dyes.

In addition to showing the course and position of fibers, Weigert-Pal preparations demonstrate whether or not the fibers have a myelin sheath. Silver chromate preparations often lead to the discovery of features of the sheaths that were not stained in earlier attempts.

Preparations stained with carmine, hematoxylin, and aniline dyes provide information on this topic as well as on the nature of cells impregnated with the Golgi method. They will also reveal cells that have not been stained by silver chromate, thus requiring further efforts to do so.

The Cox Method

Cox modified Golgi's mercuric chloride method in an advantageous way and applied it successfully to studies of the cerebral cortex. I have also used this method profitably to examine Ammon's horn and the cerebellum, and it has on many occasions allowed me to complete the information obtained with the silver chromate method.

The method can be summarized as follows:

1. Immerse fresh, relatively small pieces of neural tissue for two to three months or more in the following solution:[1]

5 percent potassium dichromate	20 g
5 percent mercuric chloride	20 g
Distilled water	30 to 40 cc
5 percent strongly alkaline potassium chromate	16 g

2. Wash the entire pieces for half an hour in 90 percent alcohol to remove excess sublimate that would ultimately precipitate as crystalline needles in the sections.

3. Mount the tissue blocks and sections as in the Golgi method.

4. Wash in 90 percent alcohol (36 percent Cartier), clean with oil of cloves, and mount with cedar oil; do not cover slip.

The Cox method, like the Golgi method, yields better results in young animals. The most beautiful preparations that I have obtained have been from the cerebral cortex, Ammon's horn, and the cerebellum of rabbits that were 20 to 30 days old. The

1. The units of measurement were omitted from the 1894 French edition, but have been included here for clarity—TRANS.

sections reveal cells and fibers that are stained with a grayish-black deposit against a yellow background.

The major advantage of the Cox method is that a large number of cells are stained without precipitates forming in superficial parts of the block. Furthermore, it readily stains the entire brain of a newborn guinea pig, as well as a one-month-old rat or mouse. The method is also valuable because the sections may be stained subsequently with Genacher carmine or with hematoxylin.

Aside from this, the methods of Cox and Golgi provide similar information. It is necessary only to bear in mind that the thinnest collaterals are more pale with the Cox method, because the metallic precipitate is less opaque than in silver chromate preparations.

Addendum

I have been led by recent studies on mammalian and chick embryos to modify slightly the diagram of horizontal collaterals that arise from the dorsal roots, as described on page 20 and the following pages.

Collaterals that arise from the principal branch and from the ascending and descending bifurcation branches differ in length and destination.

I have, in fact, observed that some of the dorsal root collaterals are long, whereas others are short.

The long collaterals arise from the principal trunk and from regions of the ascending and descending branches near the point of bifurcation. They form a dorsoventral bundle that courses radially through the dorsal horn on their way to the root cells of the ventral horn, where they end by forming a plexus around the perikaryon and dendritic processes of these cells. These collaterals form the usual pathway for reflexes, and constitute my sensory-motor pathway and Koelliker's reflexo-motor pathway.

The short collaterals arise from the remaining parts of the ascending and descending branches. They are similar to the endings of these branches in that they cross the substantia gelatinosa on their way to Clarke's column and the head of the dorsal horn, where their terminal arborizations surround various cells.

The conclusions I have drawn about the physiological significance of these observations have not changed despite this reevaluation. Weak stimuli are transmitted to ventral root cells from a limited segment of the spinal cord by way of long collaterals, while stronger stimuli also travel through the short collaterals to Clarke's column and thus to the ascending cerebellar pathway. The short collaterals also end on commissural cells in the dorsal horn, so that stronger stimuli reach from the dorsal horn to either the fundamental bundle of the lateral funiculus on the same side, or the ventrolateral funiculus on the opposite side.

Although we have not yet succeeded in demonstrating with anatomical methods a special pathway involved in transmitting sensory information over long distances to regions of the brain other than the cerebellum, the facts nevertheless dictate its existence. Thus, pathways arising from the dorsal roots are too short and do not cross the midline. This pathway appears to arise from special central sensory cells found throughout regions of the spinal cord and lower brain stem containing terminals of the dorsal root fibers. After crossing in the brain stem at the level of Reil's lemniscus or, as van Gehuchten has suggested, at the level of the ventral commissure throughout the length of the spinal cord, these axons would transmit the stimulus to the distal tufts of pyramidal cell dendrites on the opposite side of the brain.[1]

1. The reader can follow this description rather easily by simply thinking about the appropriate modifications in figures 2, 5, and 6.

Bibliography

The following bibliographic list contains only studies that are related specifically to the structure of the nervous system itself or are based on the results of new methods. I have also cited the most recent studies that have come to my attention.

General Summary

Forel: Einige hirnanatomische Betrachtungen u. Ergebnisse. *Archiv für Psychiatrie und Nervenkrankheiten*, XVIII. 5 Heft. 1887.

Cajal: Conexión general de los elementos nerviosos. *La medicina práctica*, n. 88, 1889.

His: Histogenese und Zusammenhang der Nervenelemente. *Referat. in der anat. Section des Intern. medic. Congresses zu Berlin.* Meeting on August 7, 1890.

Cajal: Réponse à M. Golgi à propos des fibrilles collatérales de la moelle et de la structure générale de la substance grise. *Anatomischer Anzeiger*, 1890.

A. Koelliker: Discours d'ouverture des sessions de la Société anatomique allemande. Munich, 1891. *Verhandlungen der anatomischen Gesellschaft.*

Van Gehuchten: Les découvertes récentes dans l'anatomie et l'histologie du système nerveux central. *Conférence donnée à la Société belge de microscopie,* April 25, 1891.

Von Lenhossék: *Neuere Forschungen über den feineren Bau des Nervensystems,* May 14, 1891.

Riese: Über die Technick der Golgi'schen Schwarzfärbung durch Silbersalze und über die Ergebnisse derselben. *Centralblatt f. Allgemeine Pathologie und pathologische Anatomie,* n. 12. 1891.

Golgi: La rete nervosa diffusa degli organi centrali del sistema nervoso. *Estratto dei Rendiconti del R. Instit. lombardi.* Ser. 2, vol. XXIV, April, 1891.

W. Waldeyer: Über einige neuere Forschungen im Gebiete der Anatomie des Centralsystems. *Deutsche medicinische Wochenschrift,* n. 44, 1891. Translated into French by Dr. Devic in *Province médicale.* 1893 and 1894.

Cajal: Siginificación fisiológica de las expansiones protoplasmticas y nerviosas de las células de la substantia gris. *Memoria leida en el Congreso médico valenciano,* session of June 24, 1891. *Revista de Ciencias Médicas de Barcelona,* n. 22 and 23. 1891.

Obersteiner: Die neueren Anschauungen über den Aufbau des Nervensystems. *Sonder-Abdruck aus der Naturwissenchaftlichen Rundschau, Jahrg. VII,* n. 1 and 2, 1892.

J. Dagonet: Les nouvelles recherches sur les éléments nerveux. *La Medecine scientifique,* pp. 11, 20, 38, 55 and 69. 1893.

V. Izquierdo: Los progresos de la Histologia de la médula espinal y del bulbo raquideo. Santiago de Chile. 1893.

Koelliker: Handbuch der Geweblehre des Menschen. Vol. 2. Elements des Nervensystems, Rückenmark, etc. 1893.

Van Gehuchten: Le système nerveux de l'homme. 1893.

L. Edinger: Zwölf Vorlesungen über den Bau der nervösen Central-Organen. 3 Auflage. Leipzig, 1892.

W. His: Über den Aufbau unseres Nervensystems. *Gesellschaft deutscher Naturforscher und Aerzte Verhandlungen,* 1893; Leipzig, 1893; and *Berliner Klin. Wochenschrift,* n. 40, 41, 1893.

Berder: La cellule nerveuse. *Thèse d'habilitation.* Lausanne, 1893.

The Spinal Cord

Golgi: Über den feinern Bau des Rückenmarks. *Anatomischer Anzeiger,* n. 13 and 14. 1890. Reproduction of an earlier study entitled: Studi istologici sul midollo spinale. *Communic. fatta al 3e Congr. freniatr. ital. tenuto in Reggio-Emilia.* September, 1880.

Golgi: La cellula nervosa motrice. *Atti del IV Congr. freniat. tenuto in Voghera.* September, 1883.

Nansen: The structure and combination of the Histological Elements of the Central Nervous Systems. *Bergens Museums Aarsberetning.* f. 1886. Bergen, 1887.

Cajal: Contribución al estudio de la estructura de la médula espinal. *Revista trimestral de Histologia,* n. 3 and 4, 1889.

—Sur l'origine et les ramificatons des fibres nerveuses de la moelle embryonnaire. *Anatomischer Anzeiger,* n. 3 and 4, 1890.

Koelliker: Über den feineren Bau des Rüchenmarks. *Sitzungsber. der Wurzb. Phys. Med. Gesellsch.* March, 1890.

Cajal: Nuevas observaciones sobre la estructura de la médula espinal de los mamiferos. April, 1890.

—Sobre la aparición de las expansiones celulares en la médula embrionaria. *Graceta sanitaria de Barcelona.* August, 1890.

—A quelle époque apparaissent les expansions des cellules nerveuses de la moelle épinière du poulet. *Anatomischer Anzeiger,* n. 21, 1890.

Von Lenhossék: Über Nervenfasern in hinteren Wurzeln welche aus dem Vorderhorn entspringen. *Anatomischer Anzeiger,* n. 13 and 14, 1890.

—Zur Kenntniss der ersten Entstehung der Nervenzellen und Nervenfasern beim Vogelembryo. *Arch. f. Anat. und Physiol. Anat. Abtheilung.* 1890.

Koelliker: Das Rückenmark. *Zeitschrift f. wissensch. Zool,* vol. LI. tt. I, 1890.

K. Schaeffer: Vergleichend-anatomische Untersuchungen über Rückenmarksfaserung. *Arch. f. mik. Anat.,* XXXVIII, 1890.

L. Auerbach: Zur Anatomie der Vorderseitenstrangreste. *Virchow's Archiv. f. pathol. Anat. u. Physiol. u. f. Klinische Medicin.* Vol. 121, 1890.

Edinger: Einiges vom Verlauf der Gefühlsbahnen im centralen Nervensystems. *Deutsch. Med. Wochenschr.,* n. 20, 1890.

P. Ramón: Las fibras colaterales de la substancia blanca en las larvas de batracio. *Gac. sanitaria de Barcelona.* October, 1890.

G. Retzius: Zur Kenntniss des centralen Nervensystems von Amphioxus lanceolatus. Vol. 2. Zur Kenntniss des centralen Nervensystems von Myxine glutinosa. *Biologische Untersuchungen, Neue Folge* 112, 1891.

M. Lavdowsky: Vom Aufbau des Rückenmarks. *Arch. f. mikros. Anat.,* vol. XXXVIII, 1891.

Claudio Sala: Estructura de la médula espinal de los batracios. February, 1892, Barcelona.

Cajal: Pequeñas comunicaciones anatómicas. La médula espinal de los reptiles y la substancia gelatinosa de Rolando. 1891.

Von Lenhossék: Beobachtungen an den Spinalganglien und dem Rückenmark von Pristiurusembryonen. *Anatomischer Anzeiger,* n. 16 and 17, 1892.

G. Sclavunos: Beiträge zur feineren Anatomie des Rückenmarkes der Amphibien. *Separatdr. aus der Festschrift zum 50 jährigen Doctorjubiläum des Hrrn Geheimrat Prof. v. Koelliker.* October, 1892.

Von Lenhossék: Der feinere Bau des Nervensystems im Lichte neuster Forschungen. 1893. Translated into French in the *Journal des Connaissances médicales,* by M. Chrétien, 1893.

Koelliker: Der feinere Bau des verlängerten Markes. *Anatomischer Anzeiger,* n. 14 and 15, 1891.

Charpy: Sur deux points récents de l'anatomie des centres nerveux. *Midi médical.* 1892.

Retzius: Zur Kenntniss der ersten Entwicklung der nervösen Elemente im Rückenmarke des Hühnchens. *Biologische Untersuchungen,* vol. V, 1893.

—Die nervösen Elemente im Rückenmarke der Knochenfische. *Biologische Untersuchungen,* vol. V, 1893.

The Cerebellum

Golgi: Sulla fina antomia degli organi centrali del sistema nervoso, 1886.

Fusari: Untersuchungen über die feinere Anatomie des Gehirnes des Teleostier. *Intern. Monatschr. f. Histol. u. Physiol.* 1887.

Cajal: Sobre las fibras nerviosas de la capa molecular del cerebelo y estructura de los centros nerviosos de las aves. *Revista trimestral de Histologia,* n. 1 and 2, 1888.

—Sobre las fibras nerviosas de la capa granulosa del cerebelo. *Revista trimestral de Histologia,* n. 4, 1889.

—Sur l'origine et la direction des prolongements nerveux de la couche moléculaire du cervelet. *Intern. Monatschr. f. Anat. u. Physiol,* vol. VI, 1889.

—Sur les fibres nerveuses de la couche granuleuse du cervelet et sur l'évolution des éléments cérébelleux. *Intern. Monatschr. f. Anat. u. Physiol,* vol. VIII, 1890.

—A propos de certains éléments bipolaires du cervelet avec quelques détails nouveaux sur l'évolution des fibres cérébelleuses. *Intern. Monatschrift f. Anat. u. Phys.,* vol. VII, 1890.

Koelliker: Zur feineren Anatomie des centralen Nervensystems. Erster Beitrag. Das Kleinhirn. *Zeitschrift f. wiss. Zool,* vol. 49. H. 4, 1890.

P. Ramón: Notas preventivas sobre la estructura de los centros nerviosos. III. Estructura del cerebelo de los peces. *Gaceta san. de Barcelona,* N. 1, 1890.

Van Gehuchten: La structure des centres nerveux: la moelle épinière et le cervelet. *La Cellule,* vol. VI. 2 fasc. 1890.

G. Retzius: Über den Bau der Oberflächenschichte der Grosshirnrinde beim Menchen und bei den Säugethieren. *Biologiska Föreningens Forhandlingar,* 1891.

Von Lenhossék: Demonstrations faites dans les sessions du 18 au 20 mai 1891, à la Société anatomique allemande. Munich.

G. Retzius: Die nervösen Elemente der Kleinhirnrinde, 1892. *Biologische Untersuchungen,* new series III, 2.

Schaper: Zur feineren Anatomie des Kleinhirns der Teleostier. *Anatomischer Anzeiger,* n. 21 and 22, 1893.

Retzius: Über die Golgi'schen Zellen und die Kletterfasern Ramon y Cajal's in der Kleinhirnrinde. *Biologische Untersuchungen,* new series IV, 1892.

Cesar Falcone: La corteccia del cervelletto. Naples, 1893.

H.-J. Berkley: The cerebellar cortex of the Dog. Baltimore, 1893. (This author does not seem to be acquainted with the works of Golgi, Koelliker and Cajal on this subject).

L. Azoulay: Quelques particularités de la structure du cervelet chez l'enfant. Société anatomique et Soc. de biologie. March, 1894.

The Cerebral Cortex

Golgi: Sulla fina anatomia degli organi centrali del sistema nervoso. 1886.

Mondino: Ricerche macro-microscopiche sui centri nervosi. Turin, 1887.

Flechsig: Über eine neue Färbungsmethode des centralen Nervensystems, etc. *Arch. f. Anat. u. Physiol. Abtheilung,* 5 and 6, 1889.

Oyarzum: Über den feineren Bau des Vorderhirns der Amphibien. *Arch. f. mik. Anat.*, vol. XXXIV, 1889.

Martinotti: Contributo allo Studio della corteccia cerebrale ed all' origine dei nervi. *Annali di freniatria e scienze affini del R. Manicomio di Torino*, 1889, and *Internationale Monatschrift f. Anat. und Physiol.*, vol. VII, 2, 1890.

Cajal: Textura de las circunvoluciones cerebrales de los mamiferos inferiores. November, 1890.

—Sobre la existencia de celulas nerviosas especiales en la primera capa de las circonvoluciones cerebrales. *Gaceta médica catalana*. November, 1890.

—Sobre la existencia de bifurcaciones y colaterales en los nervios sensitivos craneales y substancia blanca del cerebro. *Gaceta saniteria de Barcelona*. April, 1891.

—Sobre la existencia de colaterales y bifurcaciones en la substancia blanca de la corteza gris del cerebro. (Pequeñas communicaciones anatómicas). December, 1890.

—Sur la structure de l'écorce cérébrale de quelques mammifères. *La Cellule*, vol. VII, I, 1891.

—Pequeñas contribuciones al conocimiento del sistema nervioso. II. Estructura fundamental de la corteza cerebral de los batracios, reptiles y aves. August, 1891.

Pedro Ramón: El encéfalo de los reptiles. September, 1891.

Cajal: Estructura de la corteza occipital inferior. *Anales de la Soc. esp. de Historia natural.*, series II. vol. I, IV., 1893.

Andriezen: On a system of fibre-cells surrounding the blood-vessels of the Brain of Man, etc. *Intern. Monatschrift f. Anat. u. Physiol.*, vol. X, 1893.

Cajal: Beiträge zur feineren Anatomie des grossen Hirns.—I. Über feinere Struktur des Ammonshornes.—II. Über den Bau der Binde des unteren Hinterhauptslappens der kleinen Säugethiere. *Zeitschr. f. wissensch. Zool.* vol. LVI, 4. 1893.

Calleja: La region olfatoria del cerebro. Madrid, 1893.

Sala Pons: La corteza cerebral de los aves. Madrid, 1893. Résumé la *Société de Biologie*, December, 1893.

P. Fish: The indusium of the callosum. *Journ. of comparative Neurology*. Cincinnati. 1893.

Retzius: Die Cajal'sche Zellen der Grosshirnrinde beim Menschen und bei Säugethieren. *Biologische Untersuchungen.*, vol. V.

A. Thomas: Contribution l'étude de l'évolution des cellules cérébrales par la méthode de Golgi. *Société de Biologie*, January 27, 1894.

Ammon's Horn and the Fascia Dentata

Golgi: Sulla fina anatomia degli organi centrali del sistema nervoso. Milan, 1886.

L. Sala: Zur feineren Anatomie des grossen Seepferdefusses. *Zeitschr. f. wissenchaft. Zool.*, LII, I, 1891.

K. Schaeffer: Beitrag zur Histologie der Ammonshornformation. *Arch. f. mik. Anat.*, vol. 39, 4., 1892.

Cajal: Observaciónes anatomicas sobre la corteza cerebral y asta de Ammon. *Actas de la Sociedad española de Historia natural*, 2d. series, vol. 2, December, 1892.

—Estructura del asta de Ammon con 16 figuras. *Anales de la Sociedad española de historia natural.*, 2d. series, vol. I, 4, 1893.

L. Azoulay: La corne d'Ammon chez l'homme. *Société anatomique*, January, 1894, and *Société de Biologie*, March, 1894.

Olfactory Bulb

Golgi: Sulla fina struttura dei Bulbi olfatorii. Reggio Emilia, 1875.

W. His: Die Formentwickelung des menschlichen Vorderhirns vom Ende des ersten bis zum Beginn des dritten Monats. *Des XV. Bandes der Abhandl. d. math.-phys.-class. der Königl. Sächsischen Gessellch. d. Wissensch.*, n. VIII., 1889.

P. Ramón: Estructura de los bulbos olfatorios de las aves. *Gaceta sanitaria de Barcelona.* July, 1890.

Cajal: Origen y terminación de las fibras nerviosas olfatorias. *Gaceta sanitaria de Barcelona.* December, 1890.

P. Ramón: El encéfalo de los reptiles. III. Bulbo olfatorio. September, 1891.

Van Gehuchten and Martin: Le bulbe olfactif de quelques mammifères. *La Cellule.*, vol. VII. 2, 1891.

Koelliker: Über den feineren Bau des Bulbus olfactorius. *Aus den Sitzungsber. der Wurzb. Phys.-med. Gessellschaft.* December 19, 1891.

G. Retzius: Die Endigungsweise des Riechnerven. *Biologische Untersuchungen.*, new series, III, 3, 1892.

Olfactory Mucosa

Cajal: Nuevas aplicaciones del método de coloración de Golgi. I. Terminación del nervio olfatorio en la mucosa nasal. September, 1889.

B. Grassi and Castronuovo: Beiträge zur Kenntniss der Geruchsorgans des Hundes. *Arch. f. mik. Anat.* XXXIV, 1889.

Van Gehuchten: Contribution à l'étude de la muqueuse olfactive chez les mammifères. *La Cellule*, vol. VI, 2, 1890.

Von Brunn: Beiträge zur mikroskopischen Anatomie der menschlichen Nasenhöhle. Die Endigung der Olfactoriusfasern im Jacobson'schen Organ des Schafes. *Arch. f. mikros. Anat.* XXXIX, 1892.

Von Lenhossék: Die Nervenursprünge und Endigungen im Jacobson'schen Organ des Kaninchens. *Anatomischer Anzeiger,* n. 19 u. 20, September, 1892.

Retina

Tartuferi: Sull'anatomia della Retina. *Intern. Monatschr. f. Anat. u. Physiol.* 1887.

A. Dogiel: Über das Verhalten der nervösen Elemente in der Retina der Ganoiden, Reptilien, Vögel und Saügethiere. *Anatomischer Anzeiger,* 1888.

—Über die nervösen Elemente in der Netzhaut der Amphibien und Vögel. *Anatomischer Anzeiger,* May 1, 1888.

Cajal: Morfologia y conexiones de los elementos nerviosos de la retina de las aves. *Revista trimestral de Histologia,* May 1, 1888.

—Sur la morphologie et les connexiones des éléments de la rétine des oiseaux. *Anatomischer Anzeiger,* n. 4, 1889.

Elia Baquis: Sulla retina della faina. *Anatomischer Anzeiger,* n. 13 and 14, 1890.

Cajal: Pequeñas contribuciones, etc. III. La retina de los batracios y reptiles. August 20, 1891.

—Notas preventivas sobre la retina y gran simpático de los mammiferos. *Gaceta san. de Barcelona.* December 10, 1891.

A. Dogiel: Über die nervösen Elemente in der Retina des Menshen. *Arch. f. mik. Anat.,* XXXVIII, 1891.

W. Krause: Die Retina. *Inter. Monatschrift f. Anat. u. Physiol.,* vol. VIII, 9 and 10., 1891.

—Die Retina. III. Die Retina der Amphibien. *Internat. Monatschrift f. Anat. u. Physiol.,* vol. IX, 4, 1892.

Cajal: La retina de los teleósteos y algunas observaciones sobre la de los vertebrados superiores (batracios, reptiles, aves y mamiferos). *Trabajo leido ante la Sociedad española de Historia natural en la sesión del 1.º—Junio de 1892. Anales de la Soc. esp. de Hist. nat.* vol. XXI. 1892.

—La rétine des vertébrés. *La cellule,* vol. IX, I, 1893.

Optic Centers

Tartuferi: Sull'anatomia minuta delle eminenze bigemine anteriori dell'uomo. Milan, 1885.

Fusari: Untersuchungen über die feinere Anatomie des Gehirnes des Teleostier. *Intern. Monatschr. f. Anat. u. Physiol.* 1887.

Cajal: Estructura del lóbulo óptico de las aves y origen de los nervios ópticos de los vertebrados. *Revista trimestral de Histol.,* n. 3 and 4. March, 1889.

Monakow: Experimentelle und pathologisch anatomische Untersuchungen über die optischen Centren u. Bahnen. *Arch. f. Psychiatr.,* XX., 3., 1889.

P. Ramón: Investigaciones de histologia comparada en los centros ópticos de los vertebrados. Doctoral Thesis, Madrid, 1890.

—El encéfalo de los reptiles. 1891.

—Notas preventivas sobre la estructura de los centros nerviosos. I. Terminación del nervio óptico en los cuerpos geniculados y tubérculos cuadrigéminos. *Gaz. sanit. de Barcelona.* September, 1890.

Cajal: Sur la fine structure du lobe optique des oiseaux et sur l'origine réele des nerfs optiques: *Intern. Monatschr. f. Anat. u. Physiol.*, vol. VIII, 9 and 10., 1891.

Van Gehuchten: La structure des lobes optiques de l'embryon de poulet. *La cellule.* vol. VIII, fasc. I, 1892.

Sensory Ganglia and Endings (Hearing, etc.)

His: Zur Geschichte des menschlichen Rückenmarkes und der Nervenwurzeln. *Abhandl. der Math. phys. Classe d. Kais. Sächs. Gesell. d. Wissensch.*, vol. XIII, n. VI, 1886.

Von Lenhossék: Untersuchungen über die Spinalganglien des Frosches. *Arch. f. mik. Anat.*, vol. 26, 1886.

Ehrlich: Über die Methylenblaureaction der lebenden Nervensubstanz. *Deutch. med. Wochenschrift*, n. 4, 1886.

G. Retzius: Zur Kenntniss der Ganglienzellen des Sympathicus. *Biologiska Föreningens Forhandlingar*, vol. II. n. 1–2, November, 1889.

C. Arnstein: Die Methylenfärbung als histologische Methode. *Anatomischer Anzeiger*, vol. II. n. 5, 1887.

G. Retzius: Zur Kenntniss des Nervensystems der Crustaceen. *Biologische Untersuchungen.* New series I. Stockholm, 1890.

Cajal: Pequeñas comunicaciones anatómicas. I. Sobre la existencia de terminaciones nerviosas pericelulares en los ganglios raquidianos. Barcelona, December 1890.

—Nuevas aplicaciones del método de Golgi. II. Sobre la red nerviosa ganglionar de las vellosidades intestinales. September, 1889.

—Sobra la existencia de bifurcaciones y colaterales en los nervios sensitivos craneales, etc. *Gac. Sanit.* April 10 [*sic*].

—Pequeñas contribuciones, etc. I. Estructura y conexiones de los ganglios simpáticos (embriones de ave). August 20, 1891. Barcelona.

—Notas preventivas sobre la retina y gran simpático de los mamiferos. *Gaceta sanitaria*, December 10, 1891.

—El plexo de Auerbach de los batracios. February, 1892.

Cajal and Cl. Sala: Terminacion de los nervios y tubos glandulares del páncreas de los vertebrados, etc. December 28, 1891.

W. Biedermann: Über den Ursprung und die Endigungsweisse der Nerven in den Ganglien wirbelloser Thiere. *Jenaische Zeitchrift f. Naturwissenschaften.* vol. 29, 1891.

Von Lenhossék: Ursprung, Verlauf und Endigung der sensibeln Nervenfasern beim Lumbricus. *Arch. f. mikros. Anat.,* vol. 39, 1892.

G. Retzius: Über den Typus der sympathischen Ganglienzellen der höheren Thiere. *Biologische Untersuchungen.* New series III.

—Zur Kenntniss des Nervensystems der Crustaceen. *Biologische Untersuchungen.* New series I, 1890. Zur Kenntniss des centralen Nervensystems des Wurmes. Neue Folge II, 1891. Das Nervensystem der Lumbricinen. New series III, 1892.

Van Gehuchten: Contribution à l'étude des ganglions cérébro-spinaux. *La Cellule,* vol. VIII, 2, June, 1892.

—Nouvelles recherches sur les ganglions cérébro-spinaux. *La Cellule,* vol. VIII, 2, August, 1892.

—Les cellules nerveuses du sympathique chez quelques mammifères et chez l'homme. *La Cellule,* vol. VIII, 1, 1892.

Luigi Sala: Sulla fina anatomia dei ganglii del simpatico. (Note). *Monitore zoologico italiano.* III, n. 7–8, August 31, 1892.

Von Lenhossék: Beobachtungen an den Spinalganglien u. dem Rückenmark von Pristiurus Embryonen. *Anat. Anz.,* vol. VII, n. 16–17, 1892.

Erik Müller: Zur Kenntniss der Ausbreitung und Endigungsweise der Magen-Darm- und Pancreas-Nerven. *Arch. f. mik. Anat.,* vol. XL, 3, 1892.

Berkley: The nerves and nerve endings of the mucous layer of the ileum, etc. *Anatomischer Anzeiger,* vol. VIII. n. 1, 1893.

Cajal: Los ganglios y plexos nerviosos del intestino de los mamiferos. *Résumé à la Société de Biologie.* Madrid, December, 1893.

Von Lenhossék: Die Nervenendigungen in den Maculae und cristae acusticae. Special issue of *Anatomischen Heften.* Edited by F. Merkel and Bonnet.

F. Mall: Histogenesis of the retina in Amblystoma and Necturus. *Journal of Morphology.* Vol. VIII. n. 2. Boston, 1893. (This author does not seem to be acquainted with Cajal's study, La rétine des vertébrés, *La Cellule,* 1892).

Van Gehuchten: Les nerfs des poils. Brussells, 1893.

G. Sclavunos: Über die feineren Nerven und ihre Endigungen in den männlichen Genitalien. *Anatomischer Anzeiger,* n. 1 u. 2, 1893.

Retzius: Weiteres über die Endigungsweise des Gehörnerven. Biologischen Untersuchungen, vol. V, 1893.

Neuroglia

Golgi: Sulla fina anatomia degli organi centrali del sistema nervoso. Milan, 1885.

Petrone: Intorno allo studio della struttura della neuroglia dei centri nervosi cerebrospinali. *Gaz. degli Ospitali.* 1887.

Magini: Neuroglia e cellule nervose cerebrali nei feti. *Atti dell XII Congresso medico.* Pavia, 1888.

Falzacappa: Genesi della cellula nervosa e intima struttura del sistema centrale nervoso degli uccelli. *Bolet. della società di naturalisti in Napoli,* Ser. I, vol. II, 1888.

Cajal: See his Memoirs, especially on the spinal cord, brain and cerebellum. *Anatomischer Anzeiger,* n. 3 y 4, 1890, and *Revista trimestral de Histol.,* n. 3 y 4. 1889. Pequeñas contribuciones al conocimiento del sistema nervioso. August, 1891, etc.

Lachi: Contributo alla istogenesi della neuroglia nel midollo spinale del pollo. Pisa, 1890.

Koelliker: Das Rückenmark. *Zeitschr. f. wissensch. Zool.,* LI, 1, 1890.

Retzius: Zur Kenntniss der Ependymzellen der Centralorgane. *Verhandl. d. Biologisch. Vereins.* 1891.

—Zur Kenntniss des centralen Nervensystems von Myxine glutinosa. *Biologische Untersuchungen,* new series II, 1891.

Von Lenhossék: Zur Kenntniss der Neuroglia des menschlichen Rückenmarks. *Verhandl. d. anatomisch. Gesellschaft.* 18–20 Mai, 1891.

Cl. Sala: Estructura de la médula espinal de los batracios. February, 1892.

Retzius: Studien über Ependym und Neuroglia. *Biologische Untersuchungen.* New series, 1893.

F.-P. De Bono: Sulla nevroglia del nervo ottico e del chiasma in taluni vertebrati. *Communicazione preventiva al XIII Congresso dell'Associazione ottalmologica italiana in Palermo,* 1892; *Archivio di ottalmologia,* 1893.

L. Azoulay: L'origine et l'aspect des cellules de la névroglie dans les centres nerveux de l'enfant. *Soc. anat. et de biologie.* March, 1894.

Appendix A
Preface to the 1894 Edition

Anatomical studies of the nervous system are particularly concerned with physiological implications. The highest, most complex functions must be addressed, and descriptive anatomy, which has illuminated many facets of muscle and joint physiology adequately, provides little information about the possible function of conductors and nerve centers. Anatomy only began to provide a foundation for physiological insights when ideas derived from histology were combined with a knowledge of the basic elements, cells and nerve fibers. From this has emerged the concept of the reflex act and its components, the centripetal and centrifugal conductors and the central organs, or nerve cells. Attention is now focused on these central elements. Deiters' discovery pointed to the origin of centrifugal or motor fibers; all that remained was to clarify the central connections of centripetal fibers and the relationships between nerve cells.

This problem is unique in its complexity. For example, in the gray matter of the spinal cord different sets of cells are interposed between the probable entry point of the dorsal sensory roots and the well known exit point of the ventral motor roots. In addition, different levels of the gray matter are interconnected, and share connections with the brain as well. Based on embryological considerations and the study of degenerative changes, anatomists have localized the various pathways between regions of gray matter to the white columns or funiculi. Nevertheless, the connections of these fibers, as well as the connections of the dorsal roots within the gray matter, remain to be clarified.

These connections take place in what can be described as "fundamental matter" lying between the cells that appears to consist of a fine plexus derived from the branching dendrites arising from neurons. Histologists have concentrated on this plexus for more than thirty years, although its fine, interwoven texture was impossible to study because available reagents stained all of the fibers indiscriminantly. Like untangling a skein of thread, it would have been useful to follow a single dendrite among its unstained neighbors. The study of degenerative changes relies on a technique that permits this and has revealed bundles with distinct connections and functions in the white columns.

We might also wish to reveal only a few neurons in a center, and to trace their processes and connections through the inextricable plexus, which could then be unraveled even though many of its elements are not visible. Quite unexpectedly, the Golgi method provided just such an approach, although the original method has been greatly improved with the general use of the so-called rapid method along with double-impregnation procedures. This approach has been applied by Ramón y Cajal to a variety of problems involving development of various organs. He has literally revolutionized classical ideas about the histology of the nervous system, as well as the early results of Golgi himself.

According to these classical ideas, which may be traced largely to Deiters and Gerlach, the fibrous plexus in gray matter centers consists of anastomoses between cells. For example, neural currents from the dorsal to the ventral roots were thought to pass through this fixed plexus, as well as through the cells that give rise to it. I have referred to it as a fixed plexus to indicate that the fibers join one cell to another in such a way that they are in direct continuity. And, obvious though it may be, it is nevertheless worth pointing out that the nerve cell is part of the conducting plexus that arises from it; the nerve cell body is like a large knot in the plexus. The concept advanced by Golgi was contrary to widely accepted ideas and had not been corroborated. The work of Ramón y

Cajal has provided us today with entirely new ideas that have been tested and confirmed by a number of investigators.

Golgi also reported that the axon (Deiters' process) of motor cells in the ventral horn gives rise to collaterals before myelination begins, and that such collaterals are connected with the plexus arising from other cells. He attributed a great deal of importance to this plexus. As shown in figure 2 of the present volume, this plexus is not formed by dendrites, which are characteristically thick and varicose, but instead consists of axons, which are thinner and more uniform in diameter, and divide into terminal fibers at various distances from the cell of origin. The dendrites do not anastomose with one another but instead end freely, often in contact with capillaries, so that their branches serve a nutritive role, like a root system for the nerve cell. It thus plays no role in neuronal conduction, and the cell body itself plays only a secondary role. The major function of the cell body would thus be trophic. Neural activity passes almost entirely through the reticulum of short axons and the collaterals of longer axons (see figure 2A).

The ideas advanced by Golgi failed to have a significant impact. They either remained unnoticed or were greeted skeptically because they were inconsistent with mechanisms underlying the reflex, and they reduced the nerve cell to a secondary role. However, it is important to recognize two facts among his many doubtful anatomical observations. First, with very few exceptions, all nerve cells have both dendrites and an axon. And second, dendrites do not anastomose among themselves.

Ramón y Cajal demonstrated the validity of these two conclusions, and at the same time revealed the correct nature of nerve fiber connections. Each nerve cell is in itself a tiny reflex mechanism that is excited by centripetal fibers and transmits through centrifugal or cellulipetal fibers. The former consists of the dendrites and their branches, whereas the latter is the axon and its terminal or collateral fibers. In the gray matter, transmission occurs between cells, passing from the cellulifugal processes of one to the cellulipetal processes of another, and so on, thus establishing multiple pathways. However, the communication plexus between cells is not fixed. That is, it is not based on a continuous anastomosis of fibers, but rather on the contiguity or contact of terminal arborizations between them.

These anatomical facts cannot be denied when well executed Golgi preparations are viewed under the microscope. This incontrovertible arrangement agrees completely with the physiological considerations that, as I mentioned above, dominate anatomical studies of the nervous system. Happily, Ramón y Cajal stressed this viewpoint in the closing pages of the present volume. He has even suggested (page 7) that the understanding that his work provides of the hemispheric gray matter is uniquely applicable to the problems of psychology, particularly concerning the likely histological modifications associated with brains endowed with special aptitudes, whether through heredity or as a consequence of practice and application.

It is not possible, in my opinion, to overstate the importance of the fact that transmission in the spinal cord as well as in the brain takes place by way of contiguity rather than continuity between fibers. If the fiber plexus were fixed, with intercellular connections established by way of continuity (an arrangement that could only be considered permanently fixed or established), it is difficult to understand how practice makes certain patterns of transmission underlying acts that are difficult to learn (such as writing or playing a musical instrument) so easy to perform. On the other hand, because the terminal fibers of each cell in the plexus are contiguous, neural conduction and association pathways appear to form an infinite series of switches along their course, thus clarifying how practice could accentuate transmission in certain particular directions related to particular aptitudes. The old idea of a neural plexus with preestablished, fixed connections makes the results of education difficult to understand; with contiguity between elements, I should think that the nervous system is, in a certain way, malleable.

The success of Ramón y Cajal's discoveries is based on two characteristics: their anatomical rigor and their satisfying application to physiological problems. They have enjoyed great success, in fact greater success than might have been expected on a priori grounds in an era of detailed anatomical studies on all fronts. It is true that the research of this Spanish histologist has aroused widespread interest, and that scientists in many countries have verified the results and have thus established a solid foundation for the new ideas. German scholars, who are usually so indifferent to anything they do not pioneer, were particularly intrigued with the results of the methods applied by Golgi and Ramón y Cajal, and began control experiments immediately. Koelliker played a pivotal role in this work; after writing two important papers on the cerebellum and spinal cord, he has just finished (as part of the sixth edition of his histology textbook) a volume dedicated to the nervous system in which primary attention is focused on the results of the new methods.

The influence of this work in France was equally great, although it spawned fewer control studies. I believe that I was the first to give credit to Ramón y Cajal's recent work in my course at the Faculty of Medicine in 1892. My colleague and collaborator Retterer emphasized the work even more in his lectures on histology, and at the same time we persuaded a young researcher in our laboratory, Dr. C. Conil, to attempt the Golgi method. He chose to study the olfactory bulb; and the results confirmed in all respects those of Ramón y Cajal and were published in *Mémoires de la Société de Biologie* (1892, p. 179). A series of popular articles by Professor Charpy of Toulouse and by Dagonet subsequently appeared in the *Midi médical* and *Médecine scientifique*, respectively.

However, we owe the most to Dr. Azoulay in this regard. In 1891 he undertook a study of the cerebellum and spinal cord in adult and newborn animals with the Golgi method. He has remained thoroughly abreast of Ramón y Cajal's work, and in 1893 published the Spanish anatomist's work in the *Bulletin médical*, thus providing us with an initial account of the results obtained with these methods. Thanks to his care the present volume has seen the light of day. Because of his familiarity with the procedures of the author, M. Azoulay has seen to it that they are described as explicitly as possible in this book.

It is a great honor for me to have been asked to introduce this volume to French readers. I do so with confidence because I am certain that the immense value of publishing this essentially original research will be appreciated by all. It is based on a new method; his results provide clear, accurate anatomical data that have already been widely confirmed; and these facts not only compliment classical physiological concepts but are also eminently applicable to physiological questions that remain as yet unanswered. One could not hope for more.

Even from the strictly anatomical point of view, I should like to emphasize the general value of the results obtained thus far. I have briefly alluded above to the spinal cord, and the connections of cells in the cerebellum and cerebral hemispheres will be clarified as well. And, as always, the thin neural plexuses are regarded as cellular arborizations that establish multiple contacts, but are not continuous. The same principle applies to the sense organs, and we shall pay particular attention to the fiber layers of the retina as one of the clearest examples of the power of the new method. Because of the anatomical organization of the retina, the physiological legitimacy of cellulipetal and cellulifugal processes is obvious, and the examination of peripheral elements in the sense organs lend an imposing aura of generality to the new ideas of the nervous system.

The technical procedures of Golgi and Ramón y Cajal are quite well known, having been published in all of the popular accounts and control studies. Fortunately, however, the author has decided to describe them in full at the end of this volume, providing all of the details necessary for their successful application. One may therefore hope that new researchers will follow this clear pathway, and that the new method still holds many discoveries in comparative anatomy and embryology.

But while Golgi's name will always remain associated with the method, Ramón y Cajal will be remembered as the man who opened a new era of more rational ideas about the organization of the nervous system.

MATHIAS DUVAL
March 1894

Appendix B
Foreword to the 1894 Edition

The introduction of new histological methods has led recently to remarkable developments in the study of the structure of the nervous system, particularly in humans and vertebrates. The discoveries of Golgi, Ramón y Cajal, Waldeyer, Koelliker, von Lenhossék, His, Retzius, and others cannot be ignored, and have completely altered our views about the texture and function of nerve centers.

With the goal of understanding these new ideas and affording them the greatest possible impact, I have published in the *Bulletin médical* (Paris) a French translation of an excellent summary written by Professor Ramón y Cajal of Madrid, the most brilliant practitioner of the Golgi method.

The success of this edition, which was more extensive than the original Spanish version, was greater than anticipated and led us to undertake an even larger second edition. Thanks to the extreme kindness of Professor Ramón y Cajal, I have been allowed to amend the results of some of his still unpublished studies, as well as those of other authors. Thus, in some ways this is a new work by Professor Ramón y Cajal, written in French, and considerably more complete than the German translation that appeared in Professor His' *Archiv für Anatomie und Physiologie*. It is also more detailed than the latter, which is particularly important when dealing with microscopic anatomy.

Dr. L. Azoulay
March 1894

Index